Contents

Chapter 2:
Telomeres–Nature's Clock?

Chapter 3:
Cellular Senescence and Telomeres

Telomeres and Aging

Their Roles in Cellular Senescence and Implications for Longevity

A very short introduction from
The HealthSpan Institute

The Consequences of Cellular Senescence in Tissues and Organs

Chapter 4:
Telomere Length and Organismal Aging

Chapter 5:
Implications of Telomere Shortening

Chapter 6:
Environmental and
Lifestyle Factors Affecting Telomeres

Chapter 7:
Interventions to
Support Telomere Length and Function

Chapter 8:
Ethical and Societal Considerations

Chapter 9:
The Future of Telomere Research

Conclusion

Introduction

Background on the Study of Aging and Cellular Mechanisms

Aging, a universal and multifaceted process, has intrigued scientists, philosophers, and thinkers for millennia. From searching for the fabled Fountain of Youth to modern-day efforts to combat age-related diseases, understanding the mechanisms behind aging has been a profound pursuit in both folklore and scientific communities. As advancements in science and technology have progressed, the study of aging has transitioned from mere observational accounts to deeply-rooted cellular investigations.

The question "Why do we age?" has spurred a diverse array of hypotheses over the years. Some early theories were grounded in evolution, suggesting that aging was an adaptive process to prevent overpopulation or to prioritize the well-being of younger, reproductive-age individuals. Others believed aging was the natural wear and tear on the body, a result of environmental factors and daily stressors. While both concepts hold elements of truth, our current understanding of aging is far more intricate and cellular in nature.

The 20th century heralded a new era for the study of aging. With the advent of molecular biology and genetics, scientists began to recognize that the secret to understanding aging might reside at the cellular level. Several hallmarks of aging have been identified over the decades. These include genomic instability, telomere attrition, mitochondrial dysfunction, and cellular senescence, among others. Each of these mechanisms contributes uniquely to the aging process and has its own set of implications for organismal health and lifespan.

One of the most intriguing discoveries in the study of cellular aging has been the role of telomeres. Telomeres, which are the protective caps at the ends of chromosomes, play a crucial role in maintaining genomic stability. As cells replicate, telomeres progressively shorten, a process which has been associated with cellular senescence and, subsequently, aging. The enzyme telomerase, which can replenish telomere length, is predominantly active during developmental stages but is largely dormant in adult somatic cells. The interplay between telomere shortening, telomerase activity, and cellular senescence has become a focal point of aging research.

Parallel to telomere research, other cellular mechanisms have emerged as significant contributors to the aging narrative. For instance, mitochondrial dysfunction, where the cell's energy-producing machinery becomes less efficient, has been linked to a host of age-related ailments. Additionally, cellular senescence, where cells cease to divide and function correctly, can lead to tissue degradation and inflammation, propelling the aging process.

Understanding these cellular mechanisms also casts a light on the external factors influencing aging. Environmental stressors, such as UV radiation or toxins, can exacerbate cellular damage and accelerate aging. Likewise, lifestyle choices related to diet, exercise, and stress can either mitigate or amplify these cellular aging processes. The interplay between our genes, cellular machinery, and external environment forms a complex web that governs how and why we age.

In conclusion, the study of aging has evolved significantly over the years, with a sharp focus now on cellular mechanisms. As we continue to unravel the intricacies of cellular aging, the potential to influence, and perhaps even modulate, the aging process becomes a tantalizing prospect. The study of cellular aging mechanisms, from telomeres to mitochondria, holds the promise of not just extending lifespan but, more importantly, enhancing the quality of life as we age.

What are Telomeres and Why They're Important

The complexity of our bodies is mirrored in the vast universe of our cells, with DNA as its starry constellation. Protecting the integrity of this DNA, and by extension our genetic information, are structures known as telomeres. To truly grasp their significance, it's crucial to first understand their nature and function.

Imagine the aglets at the end of a shoelace—the small, often plastic, sheaths that prevent the lace from unraveling. In the realm of cellular biology, telomeres serve a similar protective role. They are repetitive nucleotide sequences, predominantly made up of a sequence "TTAGGG" in humans, found at the termini of our linear chromosomes. These sequences, while not encoding for proteins or specific functions, play a pivotal role in safeguarding our genetic information.

Each time a cell divides, it needs to replicate its DNA so that both daughter cells inherit a complete set of genetic instructions. Due to the inherent limitations of the DNA replication machinery, the replication process cannot fully extend to the very end of linear DNA strands. This leads to a curious phenomenon: with each replication, a small portion of the DNA at the ends—i.e., the telomeres—gets omitted, leading to their progressive shortening. Without telomeres, this truncation would directly impact essential genes and lead to a loss of critical genetic information. Thus, telomeres act as buffers, sacrificing a bit of themselves to protect the integrity of the overall genome.

The importance of telomeres extends beyond their protective role. Their length acts as a sort of biological clock, marking cellular age. Once telomeres reach a critically short length, the cell perceives this as DNA damage. This triggers a cascade of cellular responses, leading the cell into a state known as "senescence" where it loses its capacity to divide. Alternatively, the cell might enter apoptosis, a programmed cell death pathway. Both these fates ensure that potential genomic instability, which could lead to diseases like cancer, is curtailed.

However, nature, in its wisdom, has also provided cells with a mechanism to rebuild telomeres: the enzyme telomerase. Telomerase can add telomeric repeats to the chromosome ends, effectively counteracting the process of telomere shortening. This enzyme is highly active during early stages of human development but is largely silenced in most adult cells, with notable exceptions being stem cells and some immune cells. The dichotomy of telomere shortening and telomerase activity forms a delicate balance, with implications for both aging and disease.

Why then, if we possess an enzyme capable of lengthening telomeres, do they shorten at all? This question underscores the complex evolutionary trade-offs at play. While longer telomeres and increased telomerase activity might seem advantageous for longevity, they also come with risks. Elevated telomerase activity can be a hallmark of many cancer cells, enabling their unchecked growth and immortality. Thus, telomere shortening can be viewed as an anti-cancer mechanism, a way to limit the number of times a cell can divide and potentially accumulate harmful mutations.

In sum, telomeres are not merely passive caps at the ends of chromosomes but dynamic entities that influence cellular fate. Their role in safeguarding genetic information, regulating cell division, and acting as indicators of cellular age positions them at the crossroads of genetics, cellular biology, and aging research. As we delve deeper into the mechanisms and mysteries of aging, telomeres emerge as both guardians of our genome and harbingers of our biological destiny.

The Central Question: Do Telomeres Hold the Key to Understanding and Possibly Mitigating the Aging Process?

Aging is a multifaceted phenomenon, a dance of genetics, environment, and time. As we've delved deeper into the microscopic realms of our biology, telomeres have come into the spotlight as potential key players in this intricate ballet. They have become emblematic of a central question in biogerontology: Can understanding telomeres provide insights into slowing, halting, or even reversing the aging process?

At the heart of this query lies the observable fact of telomere attrition with age. As aforementioned, telomeres shorten as cells divide, acting as a kind of molecular clock. When they become critically short, cells enter senescence or undergo apoptosis—both states that are associated with aging tissues. Aged tissues with a higher proportion of senescent cells tend to exhibit decreased function, increased susceptibility to disease, and heightened inflammatory responses. From a broader perspective, these cellular changes underpin many age-related diseases and conditions, from cardiovascular diseases to diminished wound healing and more.

Given this association between telomere length, cellular senescence, and aging, it's tempting to hypothesize that extending telomeres might counteract aging. Some experiments in the laboratory

14

seem to support this idea. For example, mice engineered to have increased telomerase activity (the enzyme that extends telomeres) show delayed aging and live longer. These mice appear to be protected from age-related pathologies, suggesting a link between telomere extension and increased healthspan.

But before heralding telomeres as the fountain of youth, there are essential caveats and complexities to consider. For one, while short telomeres are associated with aging, they're also protective against cancer. Shortening telomeres limit the number of times a cell can divide, thereby preventing potential malignant cells from proliferating uncontrollably. This raises a conundrum: would extending telomeres to combat aging inadvertently increase the risk of cancer?

Furthermore, aging is a complex interplay of numerous factors, and while telomeres play a role, they're just one piece in the puzzle. Other cellular processes, such as mitochondrial dysfunction, epigenetic changes, and protein aggregation, are also intimately involved in aging. Targeting telomeres alone might not address these other contributors to the aging phenotype.

Nonetheless, the allure of telomeres as therapeutic targets remains. Some researchers are exploring ways to safely boost telomerase activity or use telomere-extending agents in specific cell types or tissues, aiming to rejuvenate aged organs without increasing cancer risk. Others are investigating compounds that might clear senescent cells from tissues, an approach dubbed "senolytics." By reducing the burden of senescent cells, these therapies might ameliorate age-related tissue dysfunction and promote healthier aging.

In conclusion, while telomeres undoubtedly play a significant role in cellular aging and have potential therapeutic implications, it would be reductionist to view them as the sole key to understanding and mitigating aging. They are part of a vast, interconnected network of biological processes that contribute to the aging phenotype. Whether or not they hold the "key" to aging, telomeres certainly open a door to a deeper understanding of cellular longevity and its broader implications for human health and lifespan. As research progresses, it's hoped that the insights gleaned from telomeres will contribute to interventions that enhance both the length and quality of human life.

Chapter 1: Understanding Cellular Aging

Overview of Cellular Aging and its Biological Implications

Cellular aging, often referred to as cellular senescence, is an intricate process that underpins the broader phenomenon of organismal aging. It encompasses the myriad of changes a cell undergoes over time, leading to diminished function, altered behavior, or the cessation of cell division. To understand the scope and implications of cellular aging, we must first unravel its mechanisms and the biological consequences these mechanisms impose on organisms.

Mechanisms of Cellular Aging

At its core, cellular aging results from a combination of genetic programming and environmental damage. Several key mechanisms drive this process:

1. **DNA Damage and Repair**: Throughout life, cells are exposed to various sources of DNA damage, from UV radiation to oxidative stress. While cells have repair mechanisms, they're not flawless. Over time, accumulated DNA damage can lead to functional changes or genetic mutations.

2. **Telomere Attrition**: As previously discussed, telomeres shorten with each cell division. When they become critically short, they can trigger cellular senescence, preventing further division and altering cellular function.

3. **Mitochondrial Dysfunction**: Mitochondria, the cell's energy powerhouses, can become less efficient with age. This dysfunction

can lead to reduced energy production and increased oxidative stress, further accelerating cellular aging.

4. **Protein Homeostasis Disruption**: With age, cells can become less efficient at producing, folding, and clearing proteins. This can result in protein aggregates, which can impair cellular function and even lead to cell death.

Biological Implications

The manifestations of cellular aging have profound implications for tissues, organs, and the overall health of an organism. Some of these implications include:

1. **Tissue Degeneration and Dysfunction**: Senescent cells often release inflammatory molecules, a phenomenon termed the senescence-associated secretory phenotype (SASP). This can cause inflammation, affecting surrounding healthy cells and leading to tissue dysfunction.

2. **Increased Susceptibility to Diseases**: Cellular aging is a major risk factor for many age-related diseases. From neurodegenerative disorders like Alzheimer's to cardiovascular diseases and cancer, aged cells, with their compromised functions and increased inflammatory profile, set the stage for a myriad of health challenges.

3. **Reduced Regenerative Capacity**: A hallmark of youthful tissues is their ability to repair and regenerate efficiently. Aged tissues, with a higher proportion of senescent cells, often struggle with repair, leading to slower wound healing, and reduced recovery from injuries.

4. **Systemic Effects on Organismal Health**: The implications of cellular aging aren't limited to individual tissues or organs. The systemic release of inflammatory molecules by senescent cells can impact the entire body, contributing to chronic inflammation—a recognized driver of many age-related pathologies.

Towards a Comprehensive View

While the aforementioned mechanisms and implications provide a snapshot of cellular aging, it's essential to understand that these processes are interconnected. The aging of one cell impacts its neighbors, and the aging of one tissue can affect the function of another. The intricacies of cellular aging are mirrored in the broader context of organismal aging, with each level influencing and being influenced by the others.

In conclusion, cellular aging is both a result of the wear and tear of life and a programmed biological process. Its effects ripple outwards, from the individual cell to the entire organism, driving the aging process and determining the trajectory of health and disease. As we delve deeper into the individual facets of cellular aging in the subsequent chapters, this foundational overview will serve as a touchstone, contextualizing the broader implications of cellular senescence and its undeniable role in the tapestry of life.

Factors Contributing to Cellular Aging

Cellular aging is a multifaceted process, with both intrinsic and extrinsic factors playing pivotal roles. From the inherent vulnerabilities of our biological machinery to the external insults from our environment, various elements collectively push a cell towards its aged state. This section delves into the myriad factors that contribute to cellular aging, aiming to provide a holistic view of the forces that sculpt the life course of our cells.

Intrinsic Factors

Genetic Predeterminism: Our genetic makeup can influence our cellular aging trajectories. Some individuals carry mutations or specific gene variants that can either accelerate aging (e.g., in progeroid syndromes) or confer longevity advantages.

Metabolic Processes: The very processes that provide energy and maintain cellular functions can lead to aging. Reactive oxygen species (ROS), by-products of cellular metabolism, can cause damage to DNA, proteins, and lipids, propelling the cell towards senescence.

Epigenetic Changes: Over time, the chemical modifications on DNA and associated proteins—collectively termed the epigenome—can change, altering gene expression patterns. These epigenetic drifts can lead to decreased cellular functionality and increased susceptibility to stress.

Cellular Replicative Limits: Stemming from telomere attrition, cells have a finite number of times they can divide, known as the Hayflick limit. Once this limit is reached, cells enter a state of senescence and cease to divide.

Extrinsic Factors

Environmental Stressors: Exposure to various environmental agents, like UV radiation, pollutants, and toxins, can inflict damage on cellular components, accelerating the aging process.

Nutrition and Diet: The nutrients we consume can influence cellular aging. Both overnutrition and undernutrition can stress cells, leading to accelerated aging. Moreover, certain dietary components, such as advanced glycation end products (AGEs), can directly contribute to cellular damage.

Chronic Inflammation: Persistent, low-grade inflammation, often referred to as "inflammaging," can accelerate cellular aging. Inflammatory molecules can inflict direct damage on cells and also modulate signaling pathways that accelerate senescence.

Lifestyle Factors: Smoking, excessive alcohol consumption, lack of physical activity, and chronic stress can all expedite cellular aging. These factors often act through a combination of direct cellular damage and modulation of signaling pathways.

The Interplay of Factors

While categorizing factors as intrinsic or extrinsic offers a structured approach, it's crucial to recognize the interconnected nature of these contributors. For instance, an external factor like diet can modulate intrinsic pathways of metabolism and epigenetic landscapes. Similarly, intrinsic metabolic processes can influence how a cell responds to external environmental stressors.

Furthermore, these factors don't act in isolation. The combined stress of poor diet, exposure to toxins, and genetic predispositions can synergistically accelerate cellular aging. On the flip side, positive interventions in one area (e.g., a healthy diet) might offset negative influences in another, underscoring the potential for targeted strategies to mitigate cellular aging.

In conclusion, cellular aging emerges from a complex web of internal vulnerabilities and external pressures. Understanding these factors and their interplay is pivotal, not just for a deeper grasp of the aging process but also for designing interventions that can enhance cellular healthspan and, by extension, the health and longevity of the organism as a whole.

The Role of Genetics and Environment

Cellular aging, like many biological processes, is dictated by an intricate dance between genes and environment. These two spheres of influence mold the trajectory of our cells, determining their health, functionality, and lifespan. This section delves into the nuanced roles that genetics and environment play in cellular aging, emphasizing their individual and combined effects.

Genetics: The Inherent Blueprint

Programmed Theories of Aging: Some theories propose that aging is an intrinsic, genetically programmed process. According to these theories, genes have evolved to regulate organismal development and reproduction but may inadvertently drive aging after reproductive prime. Examples include genes that regulate growth and hormones but might promote age-related diseases in later life.

Genetic Mutations and Cellular Aging: Rare genetic mutations can significantly influence the rate of cellular aging. Progeroid syndromes, like Hutchinson-Gilford Progeria and Werner syndrome, are genetic disorders that result in accelerated aging due to specific gene mutations.

Longevity Genes: Conversely, certain genes appear protective against aging. Studies on centenarians have identified several genetic markers associated with longevity. These genes often play roles in DNA repair, metabolism, and cellular stress responses, offering insights into potential protective mechanisms against cellular aging.

Environment: The Ever-Present Sculptor

Toxins and Pollutants: Environmental toxins, such as those found in polluted air or contaminated food and water, can inflict cellular damage. Chronic exposure to these agents can cause DNA mutations, oxidative stress, and other cellular dysfunctions that expedite aging.

Diet and Nutrition: Nutrient availability and the quality of our diet exert profound effects on cellular health. Caloric restriction, for example, has been shown to delay cellular aging across multiple organisms, emphasizing the role of nutrition in modulating the pace of aging.

Stress and Hormonal Responses: Chronic stress, both psychological and physiological, can accelerate cellular aging. Stress responses often involve the release of hormones like cortisol, which, in chronic elevated levels, can impair cellular repair mechanisms and promote oxidative damage.

Physical Activity: Regular physical activity promotes cellular health by enhancing mitochondrial function, reducing oxidative stress, and facilitating cellular repair processes. Sedentary lifestyles, conversely, can promote cellular senescence and dysfunction.

The Synergy of Genetics and Environment

While it's convenient to categorize influences as genetic or environmental, it's essential to appreciate their synergistic nature. Genes can predispose an individual to certain outcomes, but environmental factors can modulate these predispositions. For example:

- An individual with a genetic predisposition for a specific age-related disease might never manifest the disease if they maintain a healthy lifestyle and avoid certain environmental triggers.
- Conversely, someone with longevity genes might experience accelerated cellular aging if exposed to chronic environmental stressors, negating their genetic advantage.

Such interplay illustrates the concept of "epigenetics"—whereby environmental factors can influence the expression of genes without altering the underlying DNA sequence. Over time, these epigenetic changes can impact cellular function and contribute to the aging process.

In conclusion, genetics provides the foundational blueprint, setting the stage for potential cellular aging trajectories. Simultaneously, the environment continuously interacts with this blueprint, shaping the actual journey of our cells through time. Recognizing the nuanced roles of genetics and environment—and their intricate interplay—offers a comprehensive understanding of cellular aging's origins and paves the way for targeted interventions to promote cellular longevity.

Chapter 2: Telomeres–Nature's Clock?

Definition and Structure of Telomeres

Telomeres, often analogized as the protective tips of shoelaces, are essential structures at the ends of our chromosomes. They play a pivotal role in preserving the stability and integrity of our genetic material. Understanding the definition and intricate structure of telomeres is crucial for appreciating their role in cellular aging and broader biological phenomena.

What are Telomeres?

At the most basic level, telomeres are repetitive nucleotide sequences found at the termini of linear chromosomes. They serve a dual purpose:

Protective Caps: Telomeres prevent chromosomes from fraying or fusing with neighboring chromosomes, which could lead to genetic instability or diseases.

Buffers Against DNA Loss: Every time a cell divides, a small amount of DNA is lost from the ends of chromosomes due to the limitations of DNA replication machinery. Telomeres act as buffers, ensuring that crucial genetic information is not eroded over successive cell divisions.

Molecular Composition of Telomeres

DNA Sequence: In humans, the telomeric DNA sequence is TTAGGG, repeated thousands of times. This sequence is bound by a specialized set of proteins, forming a protective cap over the chromosomal end.

Binding Proteins: Several proteins associate with telomeric DNA to form the shelterin complex. Key components of this complex include

TRF1, TRF2, POT1, and others. This complex not only stabilizes telomeric DNA but also regulates telomerase access, an enzyme critical for telomere maintenance.

Telomeric Loop (T-loop): To further protect the chromosome end, the linear telomeric DNA can loop back on itself to form a T-loop structure. This arrangement involves the invasion of the 3' overhang of telomeric DNA into the double-stranded telomeric repeat, forming a displacement loop (D-loop). The T-loop configuration safeguards the end of the chromosome, hiding it from DNA repair machinery that might mistakenly recognize it as a broken DNA strand.

Telomerase: The Enzyme of Telomere Maintenance

Composition: Telomerase is a ribonucleoprotein enzyme, comprising a catalytic protein component (TERT) and an RNA template (TERC). This RNA template guides the addition of telomeric repeats to the chromosome ends.

Function: In cells where it is active, telomerase counteracts telomere shortening by adding TTAGGG repeats back onto the telomeres. This is especially important in cells requiring extensive proliferation, like stem cells.

Regulation: Not all cells express telomerase. In fact, in most adult somatic cells, telomerase is inactive, leading to progressive telomere shortening over time. However, in certain cells, like cancer cells, telomerase gets reactivated, enabling these cells to maintain their telomeres and divide uncontrollably.

In conclusion, telomeres, with their repetitive DNA sequences and associated proteins, stand guard at the ends of our chromosomes, ensuring genetic stability. Their intricate structure, from the simple TTAGGG repeats to the complex T-loop formations and the protective shelterin proteins, is a testament to their evolutionary importance. Coupled with the action of telomerase, these specialized structures provide insights into cellular aging, cancer biology, and the broader landscape of genome maintenance. As we delve further into this chapter, the significance of telomeres as potential markers of biological aging becomes increasingly apparent, highlighting their promise and challenges in the realm of health and longevity.

The Role of Telomerase

Telomerase, often heralded as the "immortality enzyme," has captured the imagination of scientists and the public alike for its potential role in cellular rejuvenation and longevity. At the heart of its intrigue lies its unique ability to extend telomeres, those crucial protective caps at the ends of our chromosomes. Here, we delve deeper into the role of telomerase, exploring its function, regulation, and implications for health and disease.

What is Telomerase?

Telomerase is a specialized enzyme that synthesizes telomeric DNA sequences, counteracting the inherent telomere shortening that occurs during DNA replication. Comprising both protein and RNA components, telomerase uses its intrinsic RNA as a template to add repetitive TTAGGG sequences to the 3' end of telomeres.

Function and Mechanism of Action

Telomere Length Maintenance: The primary role of telomerase is to maintain or extend telomere length. During typical DNA replication, the end-replication problem results in the gradual shortening of telomeres. Telomerase can reverse this process by adding back the telomeric sequences, thus preserving chromosomal integrity and function.

Chromosome End Protection: Beyond simply adding sequences, the action of telomerase ensures that telomeres remain long enough to form protective structures, such as the T-loop. This shields chromosome ends from being recognized as DNA damage and prevents unwanted chromosome fusions.

Regulation of Cell Proliferation: By determining telomere length, telomerase indirectly influences cellular lifespan. Cells with critically short telomeres enter senescence or undergo apoptosis. Telomerase can potentially extend cellular lifespan by preventing telomeres from reaching this critical threshold.

Regulation of Telomerase

Cell Type Specificity: Telomerase is not uniformly active across all cell types. It is typically active in germ cells, stem cells, and certain immune cells—cells that require extensive proliferation. However, in most somatic cells, telomerase activity is low or absent, leading to progressive telomere shortening with each cell division.

Cancer and Telomerase: A significant exception to the above rule is cancer cells. Many malignant tumors reactivate telomerase, enabling these cells to divide indefinitely and evade senescence, a hallmark of cancer.

Transcriptional and Post-translational Regulation: The expression and activity of telomerase can be modulated at various levels, from the transcription of its components to post-translational modifications of the telomerase protein.

Implications for Health and Disease

Aging and Longevity: Given its role in telomere maintenance, telomerase has been implicated in aging and longevity. Short telomeres and reduced telomerase activity have been associated with age-related diseases and reduced life span in various organisms.

Cancer: The reactivation of telomerase in many cancers underscores its potential as a therapeutic target. Inhibiting telomerase in cancer cells could limit their proliferative potential. However, designing such treatments requires careful consideration to avoid unintended consequences on healthy cells.

Telomere Syndromes: Mutations in telomerase components can lead to telomere syndromes, characterized by extremely short telomeres. These conditions, like Dyskeratosis congenita, manifest with a spectrum of symptoms, including bone marrow failure and pulmonary fibrosis.

In conclusion, telomerase, with its ability to extend and maintain telomeres, sits at the crossroads of cellular aging, cancer biology, and genetic diseases. Its dual nature—as a protector of cellular longevity and a potential enabler of unchecked cellular proliferation—makes it a focal point of contemporary research. As we continue to unravel the mysteries of telomerase, we edge closer to harnessing its powers for therapeutic benefits, albeit with a profound respect for its intricate roles in cellular dynamics.

How Telomeres Shorten Over Time

Telomeres, the protective caps at the ends of our chromosomes, are dynamic structures that undergo inevitable shortening over time. This gradual erosion of telomeric DNA has profound implications for cellular aging and organismal health. But why do telomeres shorten, and what are the mechanisms driving this process? Let's delve into the intricacies of telomere dynamics.

The End-Replication Problem

Mechanistic Challenge: The very machinery responsible for DNA replication, the DNA polymerase, struggles to replicate the extreme ends of linear DNA molecules. This challenge arises from the need for an RNA primer to initiate DNA synthesis, leaving a small stretch of single-stranded DNA at the chromosome end after each replication cycle.

Consequence: With each cell division, the resulting daughter cells inherit chromosomes with slightly shorter telomeres due to this end-replication problem. Over successive divisions, this shortening accumulates.

Oxidative Stress and DNA Damage

Reactive Oxygen Species (ROS): Cellular metabolism, especially in the mitochondria, generates reactive oxygen species as by-products. These ROS can cause damage to DNA, including telomeric DNA.

Vulnerability of Telomeres: Telomeric DNA has a high guanine content, making it particularly susceptible to oxidative damage. Such damage can accelerate telomere shortening beyond the regular losses incurred during DNA replication.

Chromosome Healing and Capping

End Protection: Telomeres, in their native state, form a protective structure that shields chromosome ends from the DNA repair machinery. This prevents the erroneous recognition of chromosome ends as DNA breaks, which would otherwise lead to unwanted chromosome fusions or repairs.

Shortening and De-capping: As telomeres shorten, their ability to form protective structures diminishes. Critically short telomeres may fail to cap chromosome ends effectively, leading to DNA damage responses and activation of cell cycle checkpoints.

Telomere Attrition and Cell Fate

Cellular Senescence: When telomeres become critically short, cells can enter a state called senescence. Senescent cells cease to divide but remain metabolically active, often secreting factors that can influence neighboring cells. While this can be protective against cancer (by preventing cells with damaged DNA from dividing uncontrollably), the accumulation of senescent cells has been linked to aging and age-related diseases.

Apoptosis: In certain contexts, cells with critically short telomeres may undergo programmed cell death or apoptosis. This process eliminates potentially damaged cells but can contribute to tissue attrition and dysfunction over time.

The Balancing Act: Telomerase to the Rescue?

While the natural trajectory of telomeres is to shorten over time, the enzyme telomerase can add back telomeric sequences to the chromosome ends, potentially counterbalancing some of the losses. However, as discussed in the earlier sections, telomerase activity is limited to specific cell types, and its reactivation in somatic cells can have implications for cancer.

In conclusion, telomere shortening is a multifaceted process, driven by inherent challenges of DNA replication, cellular metabolism, and the dynamic nature of chromosome ends. While telomere attrition serves as a protective mechanism against unchecked cellular proliferation, its consequences for cellular health and function underscore its central role in the biology of aging. As the "Nature's Clock," telomeres and their progressive shortening provide a tangible measure of cellular age, reflecting the interplay of genetic programming, environmental stressors, and the passage of time.

Chapter 3: Cellular Senescence and Telomeres

The Concept of Cellular Senescence

Cellular senescence, a state where cells lose their ability to divide and function optimally, has emerged as a central concept in the study of aging and age-related diseases. While initially recognized for its role in tumor suppression, senescence is now understood to have a broader spectrum of physiological and pathological implications. Telomeres and their dynamics play a pivotal role in this intricate dance of cellular aging.

Defining Cellular Senescence

Cellular senescence is a cellular program that results in the irreversible cessation of cell division. Unlike quiescence, a reversible cell cycle arrest, senescence is a terminal state. Cells that undergo senescence can remain metabolically active but exhibit changes in function, morphology, and gene expression.

Triggers of Senescence

Telomere Attrition: As discussed in previous sections, progressive shortening of telomeres can activate the senescence program. When telomeres become critically short, they can trigger DNA damage responses, pushing the cell into senescence.

Oncogene Activation: An oncogene is a gene that has the potential to cause cancer. Aberrant activation of oncogenes can drive cells into rapid proliferation. However, as a defense mechanism against potential cancerous transformation, oncogene-induced replication stress can also lead to cellular senescence.

DNA Damage: Factors other than telomere shortening, such as oxidative stress or exposure to radiation, can cause DNA damage. If this damage is too severe or persistent, cells can enter senescence.

Characteristics of Senescent Cells

Morphological Changes: Senescent cells often become enlarged and flat. They may also display increased granularity.

Senescence-Associated β-galactosidase (SA-β-gal): One of the hallmark markers of senescent cells is the expression of SA-β-gal at pH 6.0. This enzymatic activity is not exclusive to senescent cells but is more prevalent in them.

Altered Gene Expression: Senescent cells show changes in the expression of many genes, including those involved in cell cycle regulation, DNA repair, and cellular metabolism.

Senescence-Associated Secretory Phenotype (SASP): Senescent cells can secrete a myriad of factors, including cytokines, growth factors, and proteases. While SASP can have beneficial effects, such as in wound healing, its chronic presence can promote inflammation and tissue dysfunction.

Physiological Roles and Implications

Tumor Suppression: Senescence acts as a barrier against cancer. By halting the cell cycle, senescence prevents the proliferation of potentially cancerous cells.

Tissue Repair: Paradoxically, while chronic inflammation driven by SASP can be detrimental, in acute settings, SASP factors can promote tissue repair and regeneration.

Development: Interestingly, senescence also plays roles in embryonic development, where it can shape structures and contribute to tissue remodeling.

Aging and Age-Related Diseases: Accumulation of senescent cells in tissues over time can contribute to aging phenotypes and the onset of age-related diseases. Factors secreted by senescent cells can drive chronic inflammation, tissue dysfunction, and promote diseases like osteoarthritis, atherosclerosis, and even neurodegenerative diseases.

In summary, cellular senescence, once merely seen as a cell's response to stress, has now taken center stage in the fields of aging and age-related diseases. The intricate relationship between telomeres and senescence underscores the delicate balance cells must strike between preserving genomic integrity and ensuring tissue function. As we further unravel the mysteries of cellular senescence, we gain insights into potential therapeutic avenues, where the modulation of senescence might hold the key to healthier aging and the mitigation of age-associated pathologies.

Telomeres and the Onset of Senescence

The complex dance of aging, with its inevitable cadence towards cellular decline, has telomeres and cellular senescence at its very core. Telomeres, the protective caps of our chromosomes, play a pivotal role in determining when a cell enters the state of senescence. But how exactly do these structures influence the onset of cellular senescence? Let's delve into this intimate relationship.

Telomeres: The Ticking Clock of Cellular Age

Function and Form: Telomeres primarily serve as genomic guardians, protecting the ends of chromosomes from being recognized as DNA breaks. This protective function is achieved through their unique repetitive DNA sequence and the specialized protein complexes that bind to them.

Erosion over Time: With each cell division, telomeres undergo inevitable shortening. This attrition, a result of the end-replication problem and other factors like oxidative stress, leads to progressively shorter telomeres as cells divide.

The Threshold of Critical Shortening

Sensing Damage: When telomeres become critically short, they can no longer form the protective structures necessary to shield chromosome ends. Consequently, these unprotected ends are recognized as DNA double-strand breaks, activating the DNA damage response (DDR) pathway.

Signaling Senescence: The DDR pathway, sensing these critically short telomeres, orchestrates a cascade of signaling events that culminate in the activation of cell cycle checkpoint proteins, like p53 and p21. This leads to a halt in the cell cycle progression, pushing the cell into a state of permanent growth arrest – cellular senescence.

Consequences of Telomere-Induced Senescence

Genomic Stability: One of the primary reasons for cells to enter senescence upon telomere shortening is to preserve genomic integrity. Senescent cells cease to divide, thus preventing the potential for chromosome fusions, rearrangements, and aneuploidy.

Senescence-Associated Secretory Phenotype (SASP): Cells undergoing senescence due to telomere shortening often develop a SASP, where they release a plethora of inflammatory and growth-promoting factors. While this can have short-term benefits, such as in tissue repair, chronic SASP can drive tissue aging and promote age-related pathologies.

Beyond the Average: Telomere Heterogeneity

Not All Telomeres Are Equal: It's important to note that not all telomeres within a cell shorten at the same rate. Research suggests that the induction of senescence may be triggered by just a few critically short telomeres, rather than the average telomere length.

Implications for Cellular Fate: This heterogeneity in telomere length implies that a cell's fate – whether it continues to divide or enters senescence – might be determined by its shortest telomeres.

Therapeutic Potential and Challenges

Telomerase and Telomere Extension: One of the evident strategies to combat telomere-induced senescence is to reactivate telomerase, the enzyme that can extend telomeres. While this has potential in regenerative medicine and age-related diseases, it poses risks, given the association of telomerase reactivation with many cancers.

Senolytics: These are a class of drugs designed to selectively eliminate senescent cells. By targeting cells that have entered senescence due to critically short telomeres, it's hoped that senolytics can ameliorate age-related tissue dysfunction.

In conclusion, telomeres play a profound role in dictating the onset of cellular senescence. Their length and integrity act as molecular switches that can determine a cell's fate, influencing tissue health and the broader spectrum of organismal aging. As we deepen our understanding of telomeres and senescence, we open doors to potential interventions that might one day revolutionize how we approach aging and age-related diseases.

The Consequences of Cellular Senescence in Tissues and Organs

Cellular senescence, once a protective mechanism against unchecked cellular proliferation and potential tumorigenesis, has broader implications when considered in the context of tissue and organ function. The accumulation of senescent cells in various tissues over time can impact not only local cellular environments but also the overall health and functionality of the organism. Here, we will explore how cellular senescence affects tissues and organs, contributing to the broader narrative of aging and age-related pathologies.

Tissue Homeostasis and Turnover

Reduced Proliferative Capacity: One of the defining features of senescent cells is their inability to divide. In tissues that rely on regular cell turnover for their function, like the skin or the intestinal lining, the accumulation of non-dividing senescent cells can impede tissue regeneration and repair.

Impaired Stem Cell Function: Stem cells are responsible for maintaining tissue homeostasis and repair throughout life. Senescence in stem cell populations can compromise their regenerative potential, leading to a decline in tissue function.

Senescence-Associated Secretory Phenotype (SASP) and Inflammation

Inflammatory Mediators: Senescent cells often secrete a myriad of factors, collectively termed the SASP. While this can have beneficial roles in certain contexts, the chronic release of pro-inflammatory cytokines, chemokines, and proteases can drive tissue inflammation.

Chronic Inflammation: The sustained presence of SASP components can lead to chronic inflammation, a key player in many age-related diseases. From atherosclerosis to neurodegenerative conditions, chronic inflammation exacerbates disease progression.

Modulation of the Surrounding Environment: SASP factors can influence neighboring cells, either pushing them towards senescence (a phenomenon termed 'bystander senescence') or altering their behavior and function.

Tissue Stiffness and Extracellular Matrix (ECM) Changes

Alterations in ECM: Senescent cells, through their secretory profile, can modify the extracellular matrix, leading to changes in tissue architecture and stiffness. This is particularly evident in aging skin, where increased tissue rigidity and reduced elasticity become prominent.

Implications for Organ Function: Changes in ECM and tissue stiffness can have profound implications for organ function. For instance, in the heart, increased stiffness can affect cardiac function and contribute to conditions like heart failure.

Potential Tumor Suppression and Promotion

Barrier to Tumorigenesis: On the positive side, cellular senescence acts as a barrier against the potential for tumor formation. By halting the cell cycle, it prevents the propagation of cells with genomic instabilities.

Tumor Promotion: Paradoxically, while senescent cells cease to divide, their secretory profile might promote tumorigenesis in surrounding cells. SASP components can facilitate a pro-tumorigenic microenvironment, aiding in tumor progression.

Organ-Specific Consequences

Brain: The accumulation of senescent cells in the brain, particularly in the astrocyte and microglial populations, has been linked to neurodegenerative diseases like Alzheimer's and Parkinson's. The inflammatory profile of these senescent cells might exacerbate neuronal damage.

Lungs: In pulmonary tissues, senescent cells can contribute to conditions like chronic obstructive pulmonary disease (COPD) and pulmonary fibrosis, affecting respiratory function.

Joints: In articular joints, the accumulation of senescent chondrocytes is associated with osteoarthritis, leading to joint pain and reduced mobility.

In essence, while cellular senescence serves critical roles in tumor suppression and tissue repair, its chronic presence and accumulation in tissues can have deleterious effects on organ function. This dual-edged nature underscores the need for a nuanced understanding of senescence in the context of aging, paving the way for therapeutic strategies that harness its benefits while mitigating its drawbacks.

Chapter 4:
Telomere Length and Organismal Aging

Studies Linking Telomere Length to Lifespan

The quest to understand the intricacies of aging and the factors that dictate lifespan has led researchers to the microscopic ends of our chromosomes – the telomeres. Over the past few decades, numerous studies have explored the correlation between telomere length and organismal lifespan, yielding insights that range from the promising to the puzzling. Here, we'll delve into key studies that have examined this connection, and what they reveal about the role of telomeres in aging.

Observational Studies in Humans

Epidemiological Insights: Numerous large-scale epidemiological studies have found an association between shorter leukocyte telomere length (LTL) and increased mortality, particularly from heart disease and infectious diseases. These studies suggest that telomere length might serve as a biomarker for aging and age-related diseases.

Genetic Determinants of Telomere Length: Genetic studies have identified specific loci associated with LTL. Individuals with genetic variants that confer longer telomeres have been shown to have a modestly increased lifespan.

Centenarians and Telomere Length: Studies focusing on centenarians, individuals who live to 100 or beyond, have yielded mixed results. While some research indicates that centenarians possess longer telomeres, others suggest that it's the rate of telomere shortening, rather than absolute length, that's more crucial for exceptional longevity.

Animal Models Provide Causative Evidence

Mice with Compromised Telomerase: Mice that are genetically modified to lack telomerase, an enzyme responsible for telomere maintenance, exhibit progressive telomere shortening over generations. These mice display premature aging symptoms and have a reduced lifespan, underscoring the importance of telomere maintenance in aging.

Reversing Aging with Telomerase: In groundbreaking experiments, researchers have shown that reactivating telomerase in mice with compromised telomeres can reverse signs of aging, suggesting a potential causal relationship between telomere length and aging phenotypes.

Birds, Telomeres, and Lifespan: Birds offer another fascinating model to study telomeres and aging. Studies on species like the European robin and the zebra finch have found that individuals with longer telomeres tend to live longer, supporting the telomere-lifespan link across different species.

Telomere Length and Healthspan

Beyond Lifespan: It's essential to note that lifespan – the sheer number of years one lives – is just one aspect of aging. Healthspan, the period of life spent in good health, is equally crucial. Some studies suggest that telomere length is more strongly correlated with healthspan than with lifespan, meaning longer telomeres might be associated with a prolonged period of disease-free life.

Cognitive Function and Telomere Length: Research has also delved into the link between telomere length and cognitive function in the elderly. While findings are preliminary, there's evidence to suggest that individuals with longer telomeres may have a reduced risk of cognitive decline and neurodegenerative diseases.

Limitations and Caveats

Correlation ≠ Causation: While many studies find a correlation between telomere length and lifespan, it's essential to approach these findings with caution. Correlation does not imply causation, and other factors might influence both telomere length and lifespan.

Interplay with Other Factors: Telomere dynamics are influenced by a myriad of genetic, environmental, and lifestyle factors. Disentangling the direct effects of telomere length on lifespan from these confounding variables remains a challenge.

In conclusion, while the relationship between telomere length and lifespan is complex and multifaceted, studies across diverse models and populations suggest a significant connection. As research continues, the hope is to unravel this relationship further, potentially unveiling strategies to harness telomere biology for healthier aging.

Impact of Shortened Telomeres on Health and Disease

The intricate dance of telomeres and their fluctuating lengths has garnered significant attention, not only because of their implications for the aging process but also for their association with various health conditions and diseases. Shortened telomeres, in particular, have been implicated in a plethora of health issues. This section delves into the impact of these minuscule DNA structures when their length is compromised.

Cardiovascular Diseases

Atherosclerosis and Heart Disease: Studies have shown that patients with chronic heart disease often exhibit shortened telomeres in their leukocytes. These shortened telomeres might reflect increased cellular aging and reduced regenerative capacity in cardiovascular tissues, increasing susceptibility to conditions like atherosclerosis.

Heart Failure: The heart's ability to regenerate and repair is critical for its function. Shortened telomeres in cardiac tissues can compromise this regenerative potential, potentially contributing to heart failure.

Neurological and Cognitive Disorders

Alzheimer's Disease: Telomere shortening has been observed in patients with Alzheimer's disease, especially in regions of the brain heavily affected by the pathology, like the hippocampus. While the causal relationship is still under investigation, telomere dynamics may play a role in the disease's progression.

Cognitive Decline: Beyond specific neurodegenerative diseases, shortened telomeres have been associated with general cognitive decline in aging populations, suggesting a link between telomere health and cognitive function.

Immune System and Infectious Diseases

Immune Senescence: The immune system's capacity to fend off infections and mount effective responses declines with age, a phenomenon termed immune senescence. Shortened telomeres in immune cells, particularly T-cells, might contribute to this reduced immune competence.

Viral Infections: Some studies indicate that individuals with shortened telomeres might be more susceptible to certain viral infections, potentially due to compromised immune responses.

Oncological Implications

Cancer Predisposition: While telomere shortening acts as a barrier against uncontrolled cellular proliferation (and thereby tumorigenesis), critically short telomeres can lead to genomic instability, increasing the risk for certain types of cancer.

Cancer Prognosis: In patients with existing cancers, telomere length in cancer cells might hold prognostic value. Some studies suggest that tumors with shortened telomeres might be more aggressive, although this relationship varies between cancer types.

Metabolic and Endocrine Disorders

Type 2 Diabetes: Shortened telomeres have been observed in patients with type 2 diabetes. Telomere shortening in pancreatic β-cells, which produce insulin, might impair their function, contributing to the disease's pathophysiology.

Osteoporosis: Bone density and health decline with age, and conditions like osteoporosis become more prevalent. There's evidence to suggest that shortened telomeres might be linked to reduced bone mineral density and increased fracture risk.

Pulmonary Conditions

Chronic Obstructive Pulmonary Disease (COPD): Lung tissues from patients with COPD often display shortened telomeres. This telomere attrition might be tied to the reduced lung function and tissue repair capacity observed in COPD patients.

Reproductive Health

Fertility and Reproductive Aging: Shortened telomeres have been associated with reduced ovarian reserve and earlier onset of menopause in women. Telomere length might serve as a marker for reproductive aging and fertility potential.

In summary, the impact of shortened telomeres reverberates across multiple organ systems and health conditions. While many of these associations are correlative, they highlight the central role telomeres might play in healthspan, disease susceptibility, and the broader narrative of human aging. As research advances, the therapeutic potential of modulating telomere length and function could open new frontiers in the fight against age-related diseases.

Challenges in Correlating Telomere Length with Aging Across Species

The world of biology is replete with complexity and nuance. While telomere length has been an exciting metric to evaluate aging processes in humans, its extrapolation to other species presents challenges. Not all organisms age similarly or even utilize telomeres in the same way. This section delves into the complexities and challenges of correlating telomere length with aging across various species.

Variability in Telomere Dynamics

Diverse Telomere Lengths in Different Species: There is a wide variation in baseline telomere lengths across different species. For instance, mice have telomeres that are much longer than human telomeres, yet their lifespan is substantially shorter.

Rate of Telomere Attrition: Even if two species have similar initial telomere lengths, the rate at which these telomeres shorten might differ significantly. A species with rapid telomere attrition might not necessarily age faster than one with slower attrition.

Different Mechanisms of Telomere Maintenance

Variable Telomerase Activity: Telomerase, the enzyme that adds telomeric repeats to chromosome ends, isn't universally active across tissues in all species. For instance, while telomerase is largely inactive in many human somatic tissues, it remains active in many tissues in mice.

Alternative Lengthening Mechanisms: Some organisms rely on alternative mechanisms for telomere lengthening, independent of telomerase. These alternative pathways can muddy the waters when trying to correlate telomere length directly with aging.

Species-Specific Lifespan Determinants

Multifactorial Nature of Aging: Aging is a multifaceted process, governed by a confluence of genetic, environmental, and stochastic factors. In some species, telomere length might be a significant determinant of aging, while in others, different factors might overshadow telomere dynamics.

Diverse Reproductive Strategies: In species with different reproductive strategies, such as those that reproduce only once in their lifetime (semelparity) versus those that reproduce multiple times (iteroparity), telomere dynamics and their relation to aging might differ.

Methodological Issues

Telomere Measurement Techniques: Various techniques, from terminal restriction fragment analysis to quantitative PCR, are employed to measure telomere length. Each has its advantages, limitations, and biases. Differences in measurement techniques can make cross-species comparisons challenging.

Tissue Specificity: Telomere length can vary across tissues within a single organism. While leukocyte telomere length is commonly studied in humans, it might not be the most relevant or accessible tissue in other species.

Evolutionary Considerations

Role of Predation and Natural Lifespan: In the wild, external factors like predation, food scarcity, or diseases often determine an organism's lifespan. Thus, the evolutionary pressure on maintaining long telomeres might differ depending on the natural challenges a species faces.

Trade-offs in Telomere Biology: Evolution often involves trade-offs. While longer telomeres might confer cellular stability, they could also raise the risk of tumorigenesis. Different species might strike various balances between these opposing pressures, affecting how telomere length correlates with aging.

In conclusion, while the study of telomeres offers a fascinating lens through which to view the aging process, its application across the vast tapestry of life on Earth is not straightforward. Each species, with its unique evolutionary history, biology, and environmental interactions, brings a different piece to the puzzle of aging. As researchers continue to dissect the intricacies of telomeres across the biological spectrum, a more nuanced understanding of their role in the aging process will undoubtedly emerge.

Chapter 5: Implications of Telomere Shortening

Telomeres and Cancer

Cancer, a constellation of diseases characterized by uncontrolled cellular proliferation, has been at the center of medical research for decades. The interplay between telomeres and cancer is multifaceted, involving a delicate balance between cellular aging and tumorigenesis. This section delves into the nuanced relationship between telomeres and the genesis and progression of cancer.

The Dual Role of Telomeres in Cancer

Protection against Cancer: At first glance, telomeres act as guardians against cancer. By inducing senescence or apoptosis when they become critically short, telomeres prevent potential cancerous cells from dividing uncontrollably. This function serves as a natural barrier against the formation of tumors.

Promotion of Tumorigenesis: Paradoxically, if cells manage to overcome this barrier (often through the reactivation of telomerase or alternative lengthening mechanisms), they can maintain or even extend their telomeres, thereby acquiring the ability to divide indefinitely – a hallmark of cancer cells.

The Role of Telomerase in Cancer

Reactivation in Cancer Cells: Telomerase, usually silent in most adult human cells, is reactivated in about 85-90% of cancers. This reactivation allows cancer cells to stabilize or even elongate their telomeres, enabling limitless replication and contributing to tumor growth.

Potential Therapeutic Target: Given its prevalence in cancer cells and its role in telomere maintenance, telomerase is being explored as a therapeutic target. Inhibiting telomerase can cause cancer cell telomeres to shorten to critical lengths, potentially inducing cell death or senescence.

Implications of Shortened Telomeres in Cancer

Genomic Instability: Critically short telomeres, if not properly capped, can lead to end-to-end chromosome fusions, creating genomic instability—a precursor to many cancer types. These genomic anomalies can give rise to mutations that drive tumorigenesis.

Influence on Cancer Progression and Aggressiveness: Some studies suggest that the degree of telomere shortening might be linked to cancer prognosis. Cancers with significantly shortened telomeres might exhibit more aggressive behaviors and poorer outcomes.

Telomeres and Cancer Risk

Predictive Value: The length of telomeres in peripheral blood cells has been investigated as a potential marker for cancer risk. Some studies have found associations between shortened leukocyte telomeres and increased risk for certain cancers, although results are varied and more research is needed.

Role in Familial Cancer Syndromes: Mutations in genes involved in telomere maintenance can lead to hereditary disorders characterized by shortened telomeres, such as dyskeratosis congenita. Individuals with these conditions often have an increased risk of developing specific cancers.

Therapeutic Implications and Challenges

Targeting Telomerase: While inhibiting telomerase activity in cancer cells seems promising, it presents challenges. Normal stem cells also express telomerase; thus, systemic inhibition might harm these essential cells.

Combination Therapies: Approaches combining telomerase inhibitors with other cancer therapies might enhance therapeutic efficacy while minimizing potential side effects.

Telomere-Based Immunotherapies: Some strategies aim to exploit the immune system's ability to recognize and target cancer cells with abnormal telomere maintenance mechanisms.

In summary, the relationship between telomeres and cancer is a complex dance of opposing forces. While telomeres and the enzymes that maintain them offer promising avenues for therapeutic intervention, a deep understanding of their dual roles in protection against and promotion of cancer is crucial. As research progresses, the hope is that harnessing the power of telomere biology can lead to novel and effective strategies in the battle against cancer.

Telomere Shortening and Cardiovascular Diseases

Cardiovascular diseases (CVD) stand as one of the leading causes of morbidity and mortality worldwide. While numerous risk factors and genetic markers have been identified, emerging evidence suggests that telomere biology, particularly telomere shortening, may also play a significant role in the pathogenesis and progression of these conditions. This section delves into the link between telomere shortening and various cardiovascular diseases.

The Connection Between Telomeres and Endothelial Function

Endothelial Senescence: The endothelium, a monolayer of cells lining the inner surface of blood vessels, plays a critical role in cardiovascular health. Telomere shortening in endothelial cells can drive them into senescence, compromising their functionality. Dysfunctional endothelium is less effective at producing vasodilators like nitric oxide, leading to reduced vessel dilation and increased risk of atherosclerosis.

Impaired Repair Mechanisms: Endothelial progenitor cells (EPCs) aid in the repair and regeneration of damaged blood vessels. EPCs with shortened telomeres may have compromised proliferative capacity, weakening vascular repair mechanisms.

Telomere Length and Atherosclerosis

Vascular Smooth Muscle Cells: Beyond the endothelium, vascular smooth muscle cells (VSMCs) also exhibit telomere shortening with age. Senescent VSMCs contribute to arterial stiffness and the progression of atherosclerotic plaques.

Chronic Inflammation: Senescent cells often secrete pro-inflammatory cytokines, a phenomenon known as the senescence-associated secretory phenotype (SASP). Chronic inflammation driven by SASP can exacerbate atherosclerotic plaque formation.

Heart Failure and Telomere Dynamics

Cardiomyocyte Renewal: While the heart has limited regenerative potential, cardiomyocyte turnover does occur. Shortened telomeres might impair the renewal of cardiomyocytes, potentially contributing to age-related declines in cardiac function.

Mitochondrial Dysfunction: Telomere shortening has been linked to mitochondrial dysfunction, which can affect the energy supply in cardiomyocytes, impacting heart health.

Telomere Shortening as a Potential Biomarker

Predictive Value: Several epidemiological studies have suggested that individuals with shorter leukocyte telomeres may be at a higher risk of cardiovascular diseases, including coronary artery disease and heart failure.

Associations with Traditional Risk Factors: Telomere shortening seems to correlate with known CVD risk factors like smoking, obesity, and hypertension. This suggests that telomere length might serve as an integrative marker of cumulative biological age and cardiovascular stress.

Therapeutic Implications

Targeting Telomerase: While telomerase reactivation has potential cancer risks, controlled and localized telomerase activation in cardiovascular tissues might offer therapeutic benefits, aiding vascular repair or slowing the progression of atherosclerosis.

Lifestyle Interventions: Factors like smoking cessation, regular exercise, and a balanced diet have been associated with longer telomeres. These interventions might provide dual benefits: directly promoting cardiovascular health and indirectly supporting telomere maintenance.

Antioxidant Therapies: Oxidative stress accelerates telomere shortening. Antioxidant therapies might help reduce telomere attrition rate, offering potential cardiovascular benefits.

In conclusion, telomere shortening and its implications in cardiovascular health have added a novel dimension to our understanding of cardiovascular diseases. By unraveling the intricate mechanisms linking telomeres to endothelial function, vascular repair, and cardiac health, we move closer to devising innovative strategies to combat the global burden of cardiovascular conditions. As with all scientific endeavors, further studies are required to translate these findings into effective and safe therapeutic applications.

Telomeres and Neurodegenerative Disorders

Neurodegenerative disorders, encompassing conditions like Alzheimer's disease (AD), Parkinson's disease (PD), and amyotrophic lateral sclerosis (ALS), are characterized by the progressive degeneration of the nervous system's structure and function. While the exact mechanisms underlying these conditions remain elusive, accumulating evidence highlights the potential role of telomere dynamics in their onset and progression. This section explores the intricate link between telomeres and neurodegenerative disorders.

Telomeres and Neural Cell Senescence

Neuronal Health: Neurons, the primary cells of the nervous system, are mostly post-mitotic, implying they seldom undergo cell division. While they were once believed to be unaffected by telomere shortening due to their non-dividing nature, recent research suggests that telomere attrition can impact neuronal health and functionality.

Glia and Telomere Shortening: Glial cells, which include astrocytes, oligodendrocytes, and microglia, play supportive roles in the nervous system. These cells can undergo cell division, and telomere shortening in glial cells may contribute to their senescence, affecting neural support and repair.

Implications for Alzheimer's Disease (AD)

Telomere Shortening in AD: Studies have shown that individuals with AD tend to have shorter telomeres in peripheral blood leukocytes compared to age-matched controls. This finding suggests systemic telomere shortening might be associated with AD risk.

Amyloid Beta and Telomeres: There is evidence that the amyloid-beta peptide, a hallmark of AD, can induce oxidative stress, which in turn accelerates telomere shortening. This cycle could contribute to neuronal loss and cognitive decline.

Insights into Parkinson's Disease (PD)

Mitochondrial Dysfunction: PD is often linked to mitochondrial dysfunction. Interestingly, telomere attrition has also been associated with mitochondrial deficits, suggesting a potential connection between telomere dynamics and PD's etiology.

Dopaminergic Neurons and Telomere Length: Some studies have explored telomere length in dopaminergic neurons, the primary cell type affected in PD. While results are mixed, understanding this relationship may offer insights into disease progression and potential therapeutic avenues.

Telomeres and Other Neurodegenerative Conditions

Huntington's Disease: This genetic condition is caused by an expanded CAG repeat in the HTT gene. Preliminary research suggests that telomere dynamics might influence the age of onset and disease progression.

ALS and Telomere Dynamics: Some studies have indicated that patients with ALS, a condition affecting motor neurons, might exhibit accelerated telomere shortening, although the implications of this observation remain under investigation.

Potential Therapeutic Approaches

Telomerase Activation: While the systemic activation of telomerase carries potential risks, like increased cancer susceptibility, targeted approaches to activate telomerase in specific neural cell populations might offer therapeutic benefits.

Antioxidant Therapies: Given the role of oxidative stress in telomere attrition and neurodegenerative disorders, antioxidant therapies might provide dual benefits by reducing oxidative damage and slowing telomere shortening.

Lifestyle Interventions: Factors like physical activity, mental stimulation, and a balanced diet, which have been associated with neuroprotective effects, might also influence telomere dynamics, offering a non-pharmacological approach to support brain health.

In summary, the nexus between telomere biology and neurodegenerative disorders presents an emerging frontier in neuroscience. As we deepen our understanding of how telomere dynamics influence neural cell health, structure, and function, there's potential to unlock novel strategies for diagnosing, monitoring, and possibly treating debilitating neurodegenerative conditions. Future research is primed to shed light on these intersections, providing hope for the millions affected by these disorders worldwide.

Chapter 6: Environmental and Lifestyle Factors Affecting Telomeres

Diet, Exercise, and Telomere Length

The intersection of lifestyle choices and telomere dynamics offers a compelling avenue for understanding the biological underpinnings of aging and disease. Diet and exercise, two central pillars of a healthy lifestyle, have shown profound implications for telomere length and, by extension, cellular aging. This section elucidates the influence of diet and physical activity on telomere biology, emphasizing the potential for modifiable factors in shaping health and longevity.

Dietary Impact on Telomeres

Antioxidant-rich Foods: Oxidative stress is a significant factor in accelerating telomere shortening. Foods rich in antioxidants, such as fruits and vegetables containing vitamins C and E, can combat oxidative stress, potentially attenuating telomere attrition. For instance, berries, nuts, and dark leafy greens are nutritional powerhouses that may support telomere maintenance.

Omega-3 Fatty Acids: Found in fatty fish like salmon, mackerel, and sardines, omega-3 fatty acids have anti-inflammatory properties. Chronic inflammation, linked to shorter telomeres, may be mitigated by regular omega-3 consumption.

Processed Foods and Telomere Length: High consumption of sugary, processed foods can induce inflammation and oxidative stress. Diets high in these foods have been associated with shorter telomeres, hinting at the potential cellular consequences of dietary choices.

Micronutrients and Telomere Dynamics: Certain micronutrients, including zinc, folate, and vitamin D, may have roles in telomere maintenance. Their dietary sufficiency can influence telomere length and cellular health.

Physical Activity and Telomere Health

Exercise-induced Benefits: Regular physical activity is known to offer a plethora of health benefits, from cardiovascular protection to improved mental health. At the cellular level, consistent exercise appears to slow the rate of telomere shortening. This protective effect may be one of the mechanisms underlying the health benefits of physical activity.

Aerobic Exercise: Activities that boost cardiovascular health, such as running, cycling, and swimming, have shown particularly strong associations with longer telomeres. The enhanced blood flow and oxygenation, combined with reduced oxidative stress and inflammation, likely contribute to this effect.

Resistance Training and Telomeres: While aerobic exercises have been studied more extensively in the context of telomeres, preliminary research suggests that resistance training, focusing on muscle strength and endurance, might also support telomere health, albeit through different mechanisms.

Balance and Flexibility: Activities like yoga and tai chi, which emphasize balance, flexibility, and mindfulness, might also influence telomere length. These effects could be mediated through stress reduction and enhanced overall well-being.

Holistic Lifestyle Approaches

Stress Reduction: Chronic psychological stress is detrimental to telomere length. Engaging in dietary and physical practices that also reduce stress, such as mindful eating or meditative exercises, can offer synergistic benefits for telomere health.

Sleep and Recovery: Adequate sleep and recovery post-exercise are crucial for overall health. There is emerging evidence suggesting that sleep quality and duration may influence telomere dynamics.

In conclusion, our daily choices surrounding diet and physical activity echo at the cellular level, influencing the very nature of our biological aging process. The interplay between what we eat, how we move, and the health of our telomeres underscores the profound potential for lifestyle interventions in promoting health and longevity. While genetics sets the stage, lifestyle choices offer an empowering avenue to shape our health trajectories, with telomeres serving as intriguing molecular markers of these decisions. As we continue to unravel these complex interactions, the age-old adage "you are what you eat" takes on renewed significance, reminding us of the intimate connection between our choices and our cellular well-being.

The Impact of Stress on Telomeres

Stress, whether stemming from psychological or environmental factors, has profound physiological effects on the body. At the cellular level, chronic stress has been linked to accelerated telomere shortening, implying that stress may be a significant player in cellular aging and associated health risks. This section dives deep into the relationship between stress and telomere dynamics, exploring the mechanistic pathways and potential interventions to mitigate these effects.

Understanding Stress-induced Cellular Damage

Oxidative Stress: One of the primary cellular impacts of chronic stress is increased oxidative stress. Reactive oxygen species (ROS) can damage DNA, and telomeres are particularly vulnerable to this assault. This oxidative damage accelerates telomere shortening, potentially hastening the onset of cellular senescence.

Inflammation and Stress: Chronic stress can also lead to systemic inflammation. Inflammatory markers, such as cytokines, have been associated with shorter telomere lengths. The combination of oxidative stress and inflammation paints a picture of a body in distress, with telomeres bearing the brunt of the damage.

Psychological Stress and Telomere Attrition

Caregiver Stress: Studies have showcased the toll of chronic psychological stress on telomeres. For instance, caregivers of chronically ill individuals, who face persistent stress, often exhibit shorter telomeres than their non-caregiving counterparts.

Childhood Adversity: Experiencing trauma or adversity in childhood has long-lasting implications for health. Research has revealed that individuals with histories of childhood trauma or persistent stressors often have shorter telomeres in adulthood.

Job-related Stress: Chronic work-related stress, whether due to long hours, job insecurity, or high demands, has also been implicated in telomere shortening. This finding underscores the systemic effects of occupational well-being on biological health.

Physiological Responses: The Role of Cortisol

Stress Hormone Dynamics: Chronic stress results in sustained elevated levels of the stress hormone cortisol. While cortisol plays vital roles in short-term stress responses, its chronic elevation can be detrimental.

Cortisol and Telomeres: Extended exposure to high cortisol levels may influence telomere length. The exact mechanisms remain under investigation, but potential pathways include increased oxidative stress and altered telomerase activity.

Potential Interventions to Counteract Stress-induced Telomere Shortening

Mindfulness and Meditation: Practices like meditation, deep breathing exercises, and mindfulness have shown promise in reducing psychological stress. Regular engagement in these practices might slow the rate of telomere attrition associated with stress.

Social Support: Building and maintaining strong social connections can serve as a buffer against the effects of stress. Positive social interactions and support systems can counteract stress-induced cellular damage.

Exercise: Physical activity, as previously discussed, can attenuate telomere shortening. It also offers a potent tool to combat stress, serving both a protective and reparative function in the context of telomere health.

In summary, the intricate dance between stress and telomere health offers a window into the profound ways our environments, experiences, and perceptions shape our cellular landscapes. While the modern world presents a myriad of stressors, understanding the biological underpinnings of these interactions empowers individuals to make informed choices. By seeking interventions that buffer against the detrimental effects of chronic stress, it is possible to support telomere health, potentially delaying the onset of associated age-related conditions and enhancing overall well-being. As research continues to expand our understanding in this realm, the promise of integrative approaches to health, blending psychological and biological insights, emerges with renewed clarity.

Other Lifestyle and Environmental Considerations

While diet, exercise, and stress are central pillars in the discussion of lifestyle factors influencing telomere length, numerous other environmental and habitual considerations play roles in shaping our telomeric landscapes. Factors such as exposure to toxins, sleep patterns, and even social connections can influence the rate at which our telomeres shorten. This section delves into these lesser-discussed, yet equally significant, influencers of telomere dynamics.

Environmental Toxins and Pollutants

Air Pollution: Chronic exposure to polluted air, particularly fine particulate matter, has been associated with shorter telomeres. These pollutants can induce oxidative stress, a known accelerator of telomere shortening.

Chemical Exposures: Certain chemicals, especially those encountered in occupational settings like pesticides or heavy metals, may have detrimental effects on telomere length. The mechanisms can range from direct DNA damage to triggering inflammatory responses.

Sleep and Circadian Rhythms

Sleep Duration and Quality: Chronic sleep deprivation or consistently poor sleep quality can lead to a host of health issues. Emerging research suggests that inadequate sleep may be linked to accelerated telomere shortening, possibly due to increased oxidative stress and inflammation.

Circadian Disruption: Our bodies operate on internal clocks, orchestrating everything from hormone release to cell repair. Disruptions in our circadian rhythms, whether due to shift work, jet lag, or other factors, might influence telomere dynamics.

Alcohol Consumption and Smoking

Tobacco Smoke: Smoking is a well-established health risk, with implications for several diseases. At the cellular level, the toxins in tobacco can cause oxidative stress, which can accelerate telomere erosion.

Alcohol: Moderate alcohol consumption has been associated with certain health benefits. However, excessive alcohol intake can lead to cellular damage, inflammation, and potentially, faster telomere attrition.

Social Connections and Loneliness

Loneliness and Isolation: Feeling chronically lonely or being socially isolated can take a toll on health. Such feelings have been linked to shorter telomeres, suggesting a biological underpinning to the health risks associated with loneliness.

Social Support: On the flip side, strong social networks and regular positive interactions can potentially buffer against telomere shortening. Social bonds might offer protection against stress, among other benefits.

Mental Health and Cognitive Activities

Depression and Anxiety: Chronic mental health conditions like depression and anxiety might influence telomere length. The physiological stress accompanying these conditions, combined with lifestyle factors often associated with them, could contribute to telomere attrition.

Cognitive Engagement: Engaging in regular cognitive activities, such as reading, puzzles, or learning new skills, might have protective effects on the brain. While the direct link to telomeres is still under investigation, cognitive stimulation could indirectly support telomere health by promoting overall well-being.

In essence, the environment we inhabit, the habits we cultivate, and the relationships we nurture all converge at the cellular level, influencing the ticking biological clocks encapsulated by our telomeres. While genetics lay the foundation, these modifiable factors offer opportunities to shape our health destinies actively. By understanding the myriad ways in which our daily lives touch upon telomere health, we can craft lifestyles that not only support longevity but also bolster the quality of our years. As the field of telomere research burgeons, it continuously underscores the intricate tapestry of biology and environment, offering insights into the holistic nature of health.

Chapter 7: Interventions to Support Telomere Length and Function

Telomerase Activation Strategies

The possibility of intervening in the telomere-telomerase system to slow down, halt, or even reverse telomere shortening has captured the imagination of scientists and the general public alike. Telomerase, the enzyme responsible for adding TTAGGG repeats to the ends of chromosomes, thus counteracting telomere attrition, stands at the heart of this interest. But how feasible is it to activate telomerase for therapeutic means? This section delves into the strategies and implications of telomerase activation.

Understanding Telomerase and Its Activation

Nature of Telomerase: Telomerase is a ribonucleoprotein complex with a unique RNA component (TERC) and a protein component (TERT). While TERC is universally present, TERT is typically restricted, explaining the limited telomerase activity in adult cells.

Rationale for Activation: As cells divide, telomeres shorten. Telomerase can counteract this shortening. Enhancing telomerase activity in cells might thus combat cellular senescence and potentially extend cellular lifespan.

Direct Activation Strategies

TERT Transcriptional Activation: Chemical agents, like TA-65, a natural compound derived from the astragalus plant, have been proposed to upregulate TERT expression, boosting telomerase activity. However, their effectiveness and safety in humans remain topics of debate.

Gene Therapy: Innovative approaches are being explored where TERT genes are introduced into cells to stimulate telomerase activity. While promising in theory, concerns about potential tumorigenesis and other unintended consequences make this a cautious avenue of exploration.

Indirect Activation Strategies

Epigenetic Modulation: Telomerase expression is also regulated epigenetically. Modifications to the epigenetic landscape might thus influence telomerase activity. Agents like the HDAC inhibitors, which modulate chromatin structure, have shown potential in this regard.

Regulation via Non-coding RNAs: MicroRNAs and other non-coding RNAs play roles in regulating TERT expression. Strategies targeting these regulatory RNAs could offer another avenue for modulating telomerase activity.

Potential Benefits of Telomerase Activation

Cellular Rejuvenation: By extending the telomeres, cells could potentially bypass the Hayflick limit, the theoretical limit to cell division, promoting tissue repair and regeneration.

Disease Delay or Prevention: Age-related diseases, particularly those where telomere shortening is a known component, might be delayed or even prevented with effective telomerase activation.

Concerns and Risks

Cancer Risk: One of the principal concerns with telomerase activation is the risk of cancer. Many tumors exhibit heightened telomerase activity, allowing them to divide uncontrollably. There's apprehension that widespread telomerase activation could inadvertently stimulate tumorigenesis.

Unknown Long-term Effects: Telomerase and telomeres are part of a complex cellular system. Modifying one component might have cascading effects elsewhere, some of which could be unpredictable.

Ethical Considerations: The idea of extending life or delaying aging brings forth ethical questions about the nature of human life, societal implications, and the potential for disparities in access to such treatments.

In conclusion, telomerase activation strategies stand at the crossroads of science, ethics, and philosophy. While the potential to slow or reverse aging is alluring, the journey is fraught with scientific and moral challenges. As research advances, a nuanced approach, emphasizing both the promise and the pitfalls, will be essential. The dream of harnessing telomerase for health and longevity remains alive, but it requires careful navigation through the intricacies of biology and the broader implications for society.

Nutritional and Pharmacological Approaches

As the knowledge surrounding telomeres and the aging process deepens, interest in interventions that could support telomere health naturally has surged. Among these interventions, nutritional and pharmacological strategies have garnered significant attention. These approaches aim to provide compounds or stimulate pathways that can positively influence telomere length and function. In this section, we explore some of the promising nutritional supplements and drugs that might impact telomere dynamics.

Nutritional Supplements

Omega-3 Fatty Acids: Found abundantly in fatty fish like salmon, these polyunsaturated fats have anti-inflammatory properties. Studies suggest that individuals with higher blood levels of omega-3s tend to have longer telomeres, potentially due to reduced oxidative stress.

Vitamin D: Known for its role in bone health, vitamin D has also been linked to telomere length. Research has indicated that individuals with optimal vitamin D levels may have longer telomeres, hinting at a protective effect.

Antioxidants: Vitamins like C and E, as well as compounds like polyphenols found in green tea, have antioxidant properties. By neutralizing free radicals, these compounds might mitigate oxidative stress, one of the factors accelerating telomere shortening.

Astaxanthin: This carotenoid, found in algae and seafood, has powerful antioxidant properties. Preliminary studies suggest it might help support telomere length by combating oxidative stress.

Polyphenols: Found in foods like berries, dark chocolate, and red wine, polyphenols have antioxidant and anti-inflammatory benefits. Resveratrol, a type of polyphenol, has been studied for its potential to activate pathways that might support telomere health.

Pharmacological Interventions

TA-65: Derived from the Astragalus plant, TA-65 is a compound believed to activate telomerase. While early studies indicated potential benefits in telomere elongation and cellular health, more extensive research is required to establish its safety and efficacy.

Rapamycin: Originally developed as an anti-fungal agent, rapamycin has shown potential in extending the lifespan of various organisms. Its influence on telomeres is still under investigation, but it might act by affecting pathways related to cellular aging and stress.

NAD+ Boosters: Nicotinamide adenine dinucleotide (NAD+) is a crucial molecule in cellular metabolism. Boosters like nicotinamide riboside (NR) and nicotinamide mononucleotide (NMN) have been explored for their potential anti-aging effects, including support for telomeres.

Senolytics: These are drugs that selectively target and eliminate senescent cells. By removing these non-functioning, telomere-depleted cells, senolytics might improve tissue function and overall health. Examples include quercetin and dasatinib.

Metformin: Commonly used for type 2 diabetes, metformin has shown potential anti-aging effects. Its impact on telomeres is still under study, but it might exert benefits through pathways like AMPK activation and reduced inflammation.

Points of Consideration

Safety First: While many nutritional supplements are generally regarded as safe, pharmacological interventions often come with side effects. Any potential telomere-lengthening benefit must be weighed against these risks.

Holistic Approach: Relying solely on supplements or drugs might be myopic. It's crucial to consider these interventions as part of a holistic approach, inclusive of diet, exercise, and other lifestyle factors.

Individual Variation: The effects of both nutritional and pharmacological interventions can vary widely between individuals due to genetics, health status, and other factors.

In sum, the realm of nutritional and pharmacological interventions offers tantalizing possibilities for supporting telomere health. As research progresses, it's essential to approach these options with an open mind, yet with due caution, considering both their potential and their limitations in the broader context of health and longevity.

Experimental Therapies and Their Potential Implications

The intrigue surrounding telomeres has spurred innovative experimental therapies that aim to rejuvenate cells, delay aging, and combat age-related diseases. These experimental approaches, while promising, are still in their infancy and come with both potential benefits and concerns. This section will delve into some of these therapies and the broader implications they may hold for medicine and society.

Gene Editing and CRISPR-Cas9

A Potential Game-Changer: The CRISPR-Cas9 system, a revolutionary gene-editing tool, has been proposed to modify genes responsible for telomere maintenance. By directly editing the DNA sequence, scientists aim to enhance telomerase activity or even extend telomeres.

Challenges: While the precision of CRISPR is its strength, off-target effects remain a concern. Moreover, the ethical considerations surrounding genetic modifications, especially in germline cells, are significant.

Telomere Extension Using RNA Templates

The Approach: Scientists have experimented with extending telomeres using RNA templates. This method involves delivering modified RNA to cells, which then elongates telomeres.

Implications: Preliminary results showed extended telomere length without increasing cancer risk in lab settings. If successful in humans, it could open doors for therapies targeting age-related diseases.

Stem Cell Therapies

Harnessing Regenerative Potential: Stem cells, known for their ability to differentiate into multiple cell types, have long telomeres. The idea is to use stem cells, or induce pluripotent stem cells, to replace aged cells in tissues, potentially rejuvenating them.

Limitations and Concerns: While stem cell therapies hold promise, challenges like immune rejection, tumorigenesis, and ethical issues related to embryonic stem cells persist.

Small Molecule Telomerase Activators

Chemical Stimulation: Apart from natural compounds like TA-65, there's an ongoing search for small molecules that can stimulate telomerase activity. These compounds could offer a more direct and potent method to counter telomere shortening.

Balancing Act: While stimulating telomerase could be beneficial for age-related diseases, there's a tightrope walk between promoting cellular rejuvenation and inadvertently promoting cancerous growth.

Implications of Experimental Therapies

Redefining Aging: If these experimental therapies prove effective in delaying or reversing cellular aging, it might transform our understanding of aging itself. Age could be perceived less as an inevitable decline and more as a modifiable condition.

Social and Ethical Considerations: The advent of powerful therapies brings forth questions of accessibility, equity, and ethics. Who gets access to these treatments? How do we ensure they don't widen existing health disparities?

Economic Impact: Effective anti-aging therapies could have profound economic implications. They could reduce healthcare costs related to age-associated diseases, but at the same time, there could be economic challenges tied to increased longevity.

Disease Management: Many age-related diseases, from neurodegenerative conditions to cardiovascular issues, could become more manageable or even preventable, transforming healthcare paradigms.

The Unknowns: With groundbreaking therapies come unforeseen consequences. The long-term effects of manipulating telomeres are still not entirely understood, and there might be risks that aren't immediately apparent.

In conclusion, the experimental therapies targeting telomeres and telomerase are at the forefront of biogerontology. They promise a future where age-related decline might be significantly decelerated or even partially reversed. However, as with all powerful tools, they come with profound questions and concerns. Balancing the potential benefits with ethical, social, and medical considerations will be the challenge of the coming decades, one that will require the collaborative efforts of scientists, ethicists, policymakers, and society at large.

Chapter 8: Ethical and Societal Considerations

Telomere research, particularly in the context of telomere extension as a potential means to combat aging, represents a thrilling frontier in biogerontology. The implications of successful telomere extension could reshape medicine, society, and even our conceptual understanding of human lifespan. However, alongside its enticing promises are profound ethical, societal, and medical challenges that must be addressed.

The Promise: Potentials of Telomere Extension

Combatting Age-related Diseases: Many age-associated conditions, from cardiovascular ailments to neurodegenerative disorders, are linked to telomere shortening. Therapies that can effectively extend telomeres might offer preventive or curative solutions for these diseases.

Extending Healthy Lifespan: More than just adding years to life, telomere extension could mean adding life to years. The prospect isn't just about longer life, but about prolonging the years of vitality, health, and productivity.

Regenerative Medicine: Shortened telomeres are associated with cellular senescence and reduced stem cell function. Telomere extension could rejuvenate stem cells, making tissue repair and organ regeneration more effective.

Economic and Social Benefits: Prolonging healthy lifespan could lead to an older but more active, productive population. This could have positive ramifications for economies, potentially offsetting some challenges posed by aging populations in many countries.

The Perils: Challenges and Concerns of Telomere Extension

Cancer Risk: The most prominent concern regarding telomere extension is the potential elevation in cancer risk. Telomerase, the enzyme that extends telomeres, is often activated in cancer cells, enabling their unchecked growth. There's a tightrope walk between promoting cellular health and inadvertently promoting malignancy.

Ethical Dilemmas: Telomere extension therapies, especially if effective, could be costly initially. This raises questions about accessibility. Who gets to avail of these treatments? Could we inadvertently widen health disparities, creating a divide between those who can afford rejuvenation and those who cannot?

Societal Impacts: If humans start living significantly longer, societal structures, from pensions to career trajectories, might need reevaluation. How would extended lifespans impact intergenerational relationships, housing, and even resources?

Overpopulation Concerns: One of the global challenges is the strain posed by an increasing population on resources, ecosystems, and the environment. If telomere extension significantly increases lifespan, it could exacerbate these challenges.

Unknown Side Effects: As with any novel medical intervention, there might be unforeseen side effects of telomere extension. The long-term impacts on individual health and potential generational effects are still unknown territories.

The Natural Course of Life: Philosophically, there's a debate about whether humans should intervene in the natural aging process. Is there intrinsic value in the life arc, with its rhythms of youth, maturity, old age, and natural decline?

Striking the Balance

The field of telomere research epitomizes the dual-edged nature of scientific advancement. On one side lies the exhilarating potential to combat age-related decline and diseases, offering a future with prolonged health and vitality. On the other side are the weighty ethical, societal, and medical challenges that such a breakthrough would introduce.

A balanced, multidisciplinary approach will be crucial. Scientists, ethicists, policymakers, and the general public must engage in dialogues, debates, and collaborations. The promise of telomere extension should be pursued with both fervent hope and grounded caution, ensuring that humanity harnesses its benefits while wisely navigating its perils.

Ethical Implications of Potential Life Extension

The prospect of life extension, especially through means like telomere manipulation, opens a Pandora's box of ethical questions. While the scientific community buzzes with excitement over the possibilities, ethicists, sociologists, and the general public must grapple with the broader implications of potentially extending human lifespan beyond natural limits.

1. The Value and Meaning of Life

Natural vs. Extended Life: Philosophical debates arise about the nature of life itself. Does intervening in the natural aging process change the inherent value or meaning of life? Is there an intrinsic rhythm to birth, growth, aging, and death that should be respected?

Quality vs. Quantity: Extending life isn't just about adding years, but ensuring those added years have value. What's the ethical stance on prolonging life if it doesn't come with quality or purpose?

2. Socio-Economic Disparities

Access and Affordability: Initially, life extension treatments could be expensive. This presents ethical challenges concerning who gets access. Will the rich live substantially longer, while the poor age and die naturally, exacerbating socio-economic divides?

Healthcare Resources: With more people living longer, there might be increased demand on healthcare resources. How do societies prioritize care? Would younger individuals with acute conditions take precedence over older individuals seeking life extension?

3. Overpopulation and Environmental Strains

Resource Scarcity: The planet already faces challenges related to overpopulation, including food and water shortages, habitat destruction, and environmental degradation. If a significant portion of the population starts living longer, these challenges could intensify.

Intergenerational Equity: Would extending the lifespan of one generation be at the expense of future generations? Ethical considerations arise about the just distribution of resources across generations.

4. Social Structures and Relationships

Family Dynamics: Longer lives could alter traditional family structures. How would relationships evolve if multiple extended generations coexist? What's the dynamic when parents live long enough to see great-great-grandchildren?

Career and Retirement: Extended working lives could become the norm. How would this impact job opportunities for younger generations? Moreover, pension systems, built on current life expectancy models, might face upheavals.

5. The Nature of Innovation

Prioritizing Research: With the allure of life extension, there's a potential for disproportionate funding and focus on anti-aging research. Is it ethical to prioritize life extension over, say, treatments for specific diseases, poverty alleviation, or education?

Moral Obligation: If the technology exists, do we have a moral obligation to use it? Conversely, if there are means to prevent disease and death, is it unethical not to employ them?

6. Personal Identity and Cultural Impacts

Evolution of Identity: How does one's sense of self evolve over an extended life? There are profound questions about personal growth, experiences, and the evolution of identity over a longer-than-natural lifespan.

Cultural Shifts: Traditions, values, and cultural norms evolve over generations. If generational turnover slows, cultural evolution might too. What are the implications of a slower-paced societal evolution?

7. The Unknowns of Playing with Nature

Unforeseen Consequences: As with all groundbreaking interventions, there could be unexpected side effects or consequences of life extension, both at individual and societal levels.

Ethical Preparedness: Are ethicists, policymakers, and societies prepared to handle the challenges introduced by life extension?

In essence, the potential to extend life is not just a scientific or medical consideration but a deeply ethical one. It challenges fundamental beliefs about the nature of life, societal structures, equity, and even personal identity. Navigating the ethics of life extension requires a collective, interdisciplinary approach, considering not just the potential benefits but also the profound and multifaceted implications for individuals and societies.

Societal Ramifications of Extended Human Lifespans

In the midst of the excitement surrounding the science of life extension, it's imperative to also anticipate and reflect upon the profound societal changes such prolonged life could usher in. While the potential benefits are many, so too are the challenges. Here we delve into some of the key societal implications that extended human lifespans could introduce.

1. Economic Structures and Impacts

Work and Retirement: With more years of vitality, retirement ages could shift. This might entail longer careers and delayed retirements. While this could mean more years of productivity, it could also lead to employment challenges for younger generations entering the workforce.

Pensions and Social Security: Current pension and social security systems operate on the premise of a set average lifespan. Prolonged life could strain these systems, demanding reformulations of benefits and potentially introducing financial challenges for governments and institutions.

2. Intergenerational Dynamics

Familial Roles: Extended lifespans mean multiple generations coexisting. The roles and dynamics within families could shift, with potentially five or more living generations. This could redefine notions of parenthood, grandparenthood, and familial responsibilities.

Cultural Exchange: Older generations traditionally pass down knowledge and values, while younger generations introduce new ideas and innovations. Extended lifespans could slow this exchange, impacting the pace of cultural evolution.

3. Education and Career Trajectories

Lifelong Learning: With longer lives might come the need for continuous education and retraining, as individuals might have multiple careers or need to adapt to rapidly changing industries.

Delayed Milestones: Extended youth or vitality could lead to delays in traditional life milestones, like higher education, marriage, or starting a family. This would impact societal norms and expectations.

4. Population Dynamics and Resource Strains

Overpopulation: One of the most discussed ramifications is the potential strain on global resources. More people living longer could exacerbate challenges related to food, water, housing, and energy.

Urbanization and Infrastructure: Cities and communities might need to adapt to accommodate a larger, older population. This could demand new infrastructure, healthcare facilities, and urban planning strategies.

5. Healthcare Systems

Demand and Allocation: While life extension aims to extend healthy years, it doesn't necessarily eliminate all health issues. Healthcare systems might face increased demands, prompting ethical questions about resource allocation.

Focus on Preventive Care: A shift might occur from treating age-associated ailments to focusing on preventive care and maintenance of vitality.

6. Societal Norms and Values

Revaluation of Age: Prolonged vitality could change societal perceptions of age, potentially reducing ageism but also introducing new complexities in how age and experience are valued.

Cultural Conservatism: With older generations living significantly longer, their cultural, social, and political influence might also extend, potentially leading to slower societal change.

7. Political and Global Implications

Elderly Influence: Longer lives could translate to extended political influence for older generations, impacting policy decisions and potentially leading to intergenerational tensions.

Global Disparities: If life extension technologies are not equally accessible globally, disparities between countries could widen, leading to geopolitical tensions and challenges.

In considering these societal ramifications, it becomes evident that life extension isn't just a matter of individual health or choice. It is a phenomenon that would ripple out, touching every aspect of society. As with all transformative advancements, collective foresight, adaptability, and a commitment to equity will be crucial in navigating the brave new world of extended human lifespans.

Chapter 9:
The Future of Telomere Research

Emerging Technologies and Techniques

The realm of telomere research has always been at the intersection of cutting-edge science and profound implications for human health. As our understanding of telomeres deepens, new technologies and methodologies have begun to emerge, holding the promise of more accurate insights, improved interventions, and broadened applications. In this chapter, we explore some of the most promising emerging technologies and techniques in the field.

1. Advanced Telomere Length Measurement

Single-Cell Telomere Length Analysis: Traditional methods provide average telomere length across a sample of cells. New techniques aim to measure telomere length at the single-cell level, offering insights into cellular heterogeneity and its implications.

High-Throughput Sequencing: Leveraging the power of next-generation sequencing allows for a more detailed analysis of telomere length and sequence variations, opening doors to more personalized approaches in telomere-related interventions.

2. Enhanced Telomerase Activation

Gene Editing and CRISPR/Cas9: The revolutionary gene-editing tool CRISPR/Cas9 holds potential in directly modifying genes responsible for telomerase production, allowing precise upregulation in cells where telomere extension is desired.

RNA-based Therapeutics: Instead of traditional small molecules, researchers are exploring RNA molecules to modulate telomerase activity. This approach might offer better specificity and fewer side effects.

3. Telomere-Protective Compounds

Drug Discovery Platforms: Advanced computational platforms and AI-driven algorithms are accelerating the discovery of compounds that can protect or even extend telomeres.

Natural Compound Libraries: There's a growing interest in natural compounds (from plants, fungi, or marine sources) that might influence telomere dynamics, with some already showing promise in preliminary studies.

4. Cellular Reprogramming

Induced Pluripotent Stem Cells (iPSCs): Techniques to revert mature cells to a stem-cell-like state (iPSCs) can reset telomere length. This might have implications for regenerative medicine, where newly generated cells with elongated telomeres can be used for therapies.

Direct Lineage Reprogramming: Bypassing the pluripotent stage, some techniques aim to convert one mature cell type directly into another, while also addressing telomere attrition.

5. 3D Chromatin Architecture Analysis

Super-Resolution Microscopy: Advanced microscopy techniques are allowing researchers to visualize telomeres and their associated proteins in the context of 3D chromatin architecture. This offers insights into how telomeres interact with other nuclear components and their role in genome organization.

6. Advanced Models for Aging and Disease

Organoids and 3D Culture Systems: Miniature, simplified organs grown in vitro (organoids) allow for a more accurate representation of in vivo conditions. Researchers can study telomere dynamics in these systems under various conditions, mimicking disease states or aging processes.

Human-on-a-Chip: Microfluidic devices integrating multiple cell types to mimic tissue interfaces and physiological responses hold promise for studying systemic effects of telomere attrition and potential interventions.

7. Integration with Systems Biology

Omics Integration: Combining telomere research with genomics, proteomics, metabolomics, and other "omics" can provide a holistic view of cellular aging. Integrated analyses can identify pathways, markers, and potential therapeutic targets related to telomere dynamics.

In summary, the future of telomere research is bright, with emerging technologies poised to expand our understanding and offer unprecedented tools for intervention. As these technologies mature and become more accessible, the possibilities for harnessing the power of telomeres in health and disease will only grow, making it an exciting time for both researchers and those hopeful for the therapeutic potential these insights can bring.

Potential Breakthroughs on the Horizon

The dynamic field of telomere research has witnessed significant advancements over the past few decades. These breakthroughs, combined with interdisciplinary collaborations, have painted a promising picture for the future. In this section, we will explore some of the potential breakthroughs that may redefine our understanding of telomeres and pave the way for revolutionary therapeutic interventions.

1. Personalized Telomere Therapies

With the advent of precision medicine, there's a growing anticipation for **individualized telomere treatments**. Leveraging genomics, researchers could potentially identify unique telomere-related genetic markers in individuals and design interventions tailored to their specific genetic makeup.

2. Synthetic Biology and Telomere Engineering

The intersection of telomere research and synthetic biology might yield extraordinary outcomes. Scientists are exploring the possibility of **constructing synthetic telomeres** that can be integrated into human cells. These custom-made telomeres could be more resistant to erosion or could interact differently with telomerase, possibly providing cells with enhanced stability or longevity.

3. The Telomere-Telomerase Feedback Loop

A deeper understanding of the feedback mechanisms between telomeres and telomerase can unlock new therapeutic avenues. Emerging research suggests that telomeres might "communicate" their length to telomerase, guiding its activity. Deciphering this feedback loop might allow scientists to **modulate telomerase activity** with higher precision, ensuring it acts only when and where needed.

4. Non-Telomeric Roles of Telomerase

Recent studies indicate that telomerase might have roles beyond just telomere elongation, including in **mitochondrial function and cellular metabolism**. Unraveling these functions could present new ways to counteract aging or age-related diseases without directly altering telomere length.

5. 4D Visualization of Telomere Dynamics

Next-generation imaging technologies are expected to provide dynamic, **four-dimensional visualizations** (three spatial dimensions plus time) of telomeres in living cells. This would offer invaluable insights into real-time telomere interactions, behaviors during cell division, and responses to various stimuli.

6. Telomere-Targeted Drug Delivery

There's budding interest in designing drugs or therapeutic agents that can **specifically target telomeres**. Such precision would enhance the efficacy of treatments, minimize off-target effects, and reduce potential risks associated with global telomerase activation, such as uncontrolled cell proliferation.

7. Cross-species Telomere Studies

While human telomere biology holds its unique intricacies, studying telomere dynamics in other organisms, especially those with exceptional longevity or regenerative capacities, can offer novel insights. Breakthroughs might emerge from understanding how certain animals, like lobsters or certain species of sharks, manage telomere attrition differently.

8. Integrative AI-driven Telomere Analysis

Advanced computational models, powered by artificial intelligence, are set to play a transformative role. These models can **integrate vast amounts of data**—from genetic sequences to cellular behaviors—to predict telomere dynamics, identify potential therapeutic targets, or even simulate the systemic effects of telomere manipulations.

9. Ethical Framework for Telomere Manipulations

As the potential of telomere interventions becomes increasingly tangible, there will be a pressing need for an **ethical framework** guiding their application. Breakthroughs in this arena will involve interdisciplinary collaborations between scientists, ethicists, policymakers, and the general public to ensure that telomere-based therapies are used responsibly and equitably.

In conclusion, the horizon of telomere research is dotted with possibilities that were once considered science fiction. While challenges remain, the combination of technological advancements, deeper biological insights, and collaborative efforts promises a future where the mysteries of telomeres are not just understood but harnessed for the betterment of human health and longevity.

Implications for Longevity and Healthspan

The study of telomeres is not merely a voyage of understanding the intricacies of molecular biology; it's fundamentally tied to the human desire to unravel the secrets of longevity and healthspan. While longevity focuses on the extension of life, healthspan emphasizes the quality of those extended years, free from age-related diseases and functional declines. As we venture into the future of telomere research, the implications for both longevity and healthspan hold promise but also present multifaceted challenges.

1. The Telomere-Healthspan Connection

It's becoming increasingly evident that telomere dynamics have pro-found **impacts on cellular health**. As telomeres shorten, cells enter a senescent state, often characterized by a loss of function and an inflammatory profile. Cumulatively, cellular senescence can manifest as tissue degeneration and dysfunction, laying the foundation for age-associated diseases. Thus, interventions that maintain or even extend telomere length have the potential to delay these detrimental processes, effectively enhancing healthspan.

2. Beyond Just Living Longer

The mere extension of lifespan without a concurrent improvement in health would be a Pyrrhic victory. The vision of the future is not just about adding years to life but adding life to years. Telomere research, by shedding light on cellular aging mechanisms, offers insights into **preserving tissue function and regenerative capacities** as we age. In essence, it's about creating an extended period of vitality, cognitive sharpness, and physical wellness.

3. A Potential Panacea for Age-Related Diseases?

Many age-related diseases, from cardiovascular ailments to neurodegenerative disorders, have been linked, at least in part, to telomere attrition. Targeted telomere therapies might offer **holistic interventions**, mitigating the risks of multiple diseases simultaneously. Instead of treating individual symptoms or diseases, the medical paradigm might shift towards treating the root causes of aging itself.

4. Complementary Therapies

The future might see telomere-based interventions not in isolation but in conjunction with other therapies. These could range from **dietary and lifestyle adjustments** that naturally support telomere health to advanced treatments like stem cell therapies or gene edits that work synergistically with telomere modifications.

5. Predictive Health Metrics

As our understanding of telomeres deepens, they could serve as **predictive biomarkers** for aging and age-related diseases. Routine assessments of telomere length and function might inform individuals of their cellular age, guiding personalized health interventions and lifestyle modifications.

6. Challenges in Achieving Extended Healthspan

It's crucial to recognize that telomeres are but one piece of the complex puzzle of aging. Other factors, from mitochondrial function to epigenetic changes, play pivotal roles in the aging process. While telomere therapies might offer significant benefits, they won't be silver bullets. A comprehensive approach to healthspan extension will likely require interventions at multiple biological levels.

7. Socioeconomic Implications of Extended Healthspan

An increase in healthspan will have ripple effects across society. On one hand, reduced medical expenses for age-related diseases could alleviate economic burdens. On the other hand, extended working lives and a shift in the dynamics of retirement, family structures, and inter-generational interactions will pose new challenges.

8. The Imperative of Equitable Access

The promise of enhanced healthspan should be a shared vision for all of humanity. As advanced telomere-based therapies emerge, it will be ethically imperative to ensure that they are not just the privilege of a few but are **accessible to diverse populations** globally.

In reflection, the future of telomere research, as it pertains to longevity and healthspan, is tantalizing. The journey ahead will be one of scientific revelations, therapeutic innovations, and societal adaptations. Embracing the challenges and opportunities of this journey could redefine our collective understanding of aging, health, and the very essence of a fulfilling life.

Conclusion

Summarizing the Current State of Knowledge and Research on Telomeres and Aging

In our journey through the realm of telomeres and aging, we have delved deep into the intricacies of cellular processes, the mysteries of longevity, and the societal and ethical ramifications of potential life extension. As we draw this exploration to a close, it's prudent to synthesize our findings and contemplate the road ahead.

1. Telomeres: Nature's Cellular Clock

Telomeres have emerged as a central figure in the narrative of cellular aging. Positioned at the ends of our chromosomes, these repetitive DNA sequences act as protective caps, ensuring the fidelity of genetic information during cell division. However, with each division, telomeres shorten—a process likened to a **biological clock** ticking away, signaling cellular age.

2. The Implications of Telomere Shortening

The shortening of telomeres is not without consequence. Once telomeres reach a critical length, cells enter a state of senescence, losing their functional capabilities and potentially secreting inflammatory compounds. This senescent state is implicated in tissue dysfunction and the onset of various age-related diseases, from cardiovascular disorders to neurodegenerative conditions.

3. Telomerase: The Enzyme of Renewal

Nature's counter to telomere shortening is **telomerase**, an enzyme capable of extending the telomeric ends. While its activity is robust during the embryonic stages, it diminishes in most somatic cells as we age. Reactivating telomerase in cells has been a focal point of research offering the tantalizing possibility of cellular rejuvenation.

4. Telomeres as Biomarkers

Increasingly, telomere length is being viewed as a potential biomarker for biological age, distinct from chronological age. Shortened telomeres have been associated with an increased risk for a spectrum of diseases and potentially reduced lifespan. Consequently, measuring telomere length could offer predictive insights, guiding individual health strategies.

5. Lifestyle, Environment, and Telomeres

Our actions and environment play a role in telomere dynamics. Factors such as **diet, exercise, and stress** have been shown to influence telomere length, suggesting that we have some agency in managing our cellular aging process. Adopting a telomere-friendly lifestyle could be a proactive approach to extending healthspan.

6. Interventions on the Horizon

Research is burgeoning in the realm of interventions, from dietary supplements to more advanced genetic and pharmacological strategies, that might support telomere health. While some are still experimental, others are already showing promise in early trials.

7. Ethical and Societal Dimensions

The potential to influence human longevity and healthspan through telomere-based interventions brings forth profound ethical questions. From the equity of access to such therapies to the societal implications of extended lifespans, the discourse around telomeres transcends biology, touching the realms of philosophy, ethics, and socioeconomics.

8. The Future Awaits

While our understanding of telomeres has grown exponentially in recent decades, it's evident that we're at the **threshold of discovery**. New technologies, evolving methodologies, and interdisciplinary collaborations promise to propel the field forward, potentially redefining our understanding of aging and the human lifespan.

In conclusion, the realm of telomeres and aging is a tapestry of molecular mechanisms, clinical implications, and societal considerations.

The confluence of these diverse threads offers a holistic view of the aging process, challenges current paradigms, and beckons us into an era where aging might be more malleable than previously imagined. The road ahead is one of promise, curiosity, and hope, and the journey promises to be as enlightening as the destination.

The Potential Promise of Telomere Research for Health and Longevity

The narrative of human existence has been punctuated by our perpetual quest to understand the underpinnings of life and, more profoundly, our desire to extend the bounds of our existence. The study of telomeres and their role in aging has emerged as a beacon in this exploration, promising insights that could reshape our understanding of health, aging, and longevity.

1. Beyond the Veil of Biological Timekeeping

Telomeres, with their repetitive DNA sequences, stand sentinel at the ends of our chromosomes. As biological timekeepers, they recede with each cell division, their waning length a harbinger of cellular age. But what if we could intervene, recalibrate, or even rejuvenate these molecular clocks? The possibility that we might influence, or even control, the tempo of this ticking has profound implications. It suggests a potential to delay or mitigate the ravages of time, ensuring not just longer life but also a longer period of good health or 'healthspan'.

2. The Intersection of Healthspan and Lifespan

While much of the dialogue around aging centers on lifespan extension, the true promise of telomere research might lie in its implications for healthspan. It's not just about adding years to life but adding life to those years. Understanding telomere dynamics could provide strategies to prevent or delay age-associated disorders, from cardiovascular diseases to cognitive decline. In essence, the focus shifts from mere survival to thriving.

3. A Paradigm Shift in Disease Management

Many age-related diseases have a common underpinning in cellular dysfunction. Telomere shortening and the ensuing cellular senescence contribute to this dysfunction. By targeting the root cause, telomere-focused interventions might offer a holistic approach to disease management, moving away from symptom alleviation to disease prevention or even reversal.

4. Personalized Medicine and Predictive Insights

Telomere length, as a biomarker of cellular age, offers a window into an individual's biological versus chronological age. This could pave the way for personalized medical strategies, wherein interventions are tailored based on an individual's telomere status. It's a step towards proactive, rather than reactive, health management.

5. Socioeconomic and Global Health Implications

Beyond individual health, the broad-scale application of telomere-centric interventions could have global implications. An increased healthspan could translate to an active, contributing elderly population, potentially alleviating some socioeconomic challenges associated with an aging demographic. On a larger scale, understanding telomere dynamics could offer insights into population health and epidemiological trends.

6. The Journey Ahead

While the promise is immense, the road to realizing the full potential of telomere research is punctuated with challenges. From the intricacies of cellular mechanisms to the ethical conundrums of life extension, the journey is multifaceted. However, with each research breakthrough, we inch closer to a future where the boundaries of human health and longevity might be more fluid than fixed.

In wrapping up our exploration, it's evident that the realm of telomeres and aging is not just a scientific endeavor but a philosophical and societal one as well. The intertwining of biology, ethics, and society offers a rich tapestry of insights, debates, and possibilities. The study of telomeres, in essence, is a reflection of our collective aspiration—to understand the dance of life, to extend its melody, and to ensure that each note, each moment, resonates with health, vitality, and purpose.

Recognizing the Complexity of Aging and the Multifaceted Roles of Telomeres

As we draw our exploration of telomeres and aging to a close, it's imperative to revisit and underline the intricate nature of the aging process and the multifarious roles that telomeres play within this intricate ballet of biology. Aging is not a singular process nor an isolated event; it is a complex tapestry woven from myriad threads, of which telomeres are but one—albeit a significant one.

1. Aging: Not Just a Cellular Event

While cellular aging, with telomeres at its core, plays a pivotal role in organismal aging, it's just one component of a vast machinery. Aging encompasses changes at the molecular, cellular, tissue, organ, system, and organismal levels. Each level is influenced by a myriad of factors—genetic, epigenetic, environmental, and lifestyle-driven. Telomere shortening and its implications for cellular senescence and function undoubtedly serve as a cornerstone, but the edifice of aging is constructed from numerous such cornerstones.

2. Telomeres: More Than Just Biological Clocks

The primary role of telomeres as protective caps for chromosomes and their function as biological indicators of cellular age is well-documented. However, their role extends beyond mere timekeeping. They are intertwined with cellular mechanisms governing DNA repair, apoptosis, and genome stability. Their length and function, influenced by a plethora of factors, from oxidative stress to telomerase activity, can also offer insights into an individual's exposure to various environmental stressors or genetic predispositions.

3. The Interplay of Genetics and Environment

Our genes set the stage, but it's the interplay with the environment that orchestrates the play of aging. Telomeres encapsulate this dance beautifully. While there's a genetic baseline for telomere length, a host of external factors—from diet and exercise to stress and environmental toxins—can influence the rate of telomere shortening. This dynamic interface between the genetic and the external is where the magic and mystery of aging truly reside.

4. The Systemic Ripple Effect

The consequences of telomere shortening and cellular senescence aren't confined to a single cell. They create ripples, influencing neighboring cells, tissues, and organs. A senescent cell, through the release of inflammatory cytokines, can influence the microenvironment, potentially promoting age-related diseases or tissue dysfunction. Thus, the localized event of telomere shortening can have systemic repercussions.

5. Embracing the Holistic View of Aging

It's tempting to seek a silver bullet, a singular key to unlock the secrets of aging. Telomeres, given their central role, often emerge as candidates for this role. However, a holistic understanding of aging requires us to view telomeres as part of an intricate puzzle. A puzzle where each piece, from mitochondrial function and protein homeostasis to hormonal regulation and neural plasticity, plays a crucial role.

6. Towards a Nuanced Understanding

As with all scientific endeavors, the study of telomeres and aging is characterized by a dance between revelation and mystery. With each finding, we unveil a layer, only to discover myriad layers beneath. It's a journey of humility, where we recognize the vastness of what we don't know while celebrating the strides we've made.

In conclusion, the narrative of telomeres and aging serves as a poignant reminder of the beautiful complexity of life. It underscores the need for a multi-pronged, interdisciplinary approach to understand, and potentially influence, the trajectory of aging. As we stand at this nexus of understanding and potential, it's evident that the tale of telomeres is not just a chapter in the story of aging but a rich, evolving subplot of its own, replete with insights, challenges, and promise.